Can You See What Eye See?

Envision a Better You and a Better World

M. CHERE SAMPSON

BALBOA.
PRESS

A DIVISION OF HAY HOUSE

Balboa Press books may be ordered through booksellers or by contacting:

Balboa Press
A Division of Hay House
1663 Liberty Drive
Bloomington, IN 47403
www.balboapress.com
1 (877) 407-4847

Because of the dynamic nature of the Internet, any web addresses or
links contained in this book may have changed since publication and
may no longer be valid. The views expressed in this work are solely those
of the author and do not necessarily reflect the views of the publisher,
and the publisher hereby disclaims any responsibility for them.

The author of this book does not dispense medical advice or prescribe the use
of any technique as a form of treatment for physical, emotional, or medical
problems without the advice of a physician, either directly or indirectly. The
intent of the author is only to offer information of a general nature to help
you in your quest for emotional and spiritual well-being. In the event you use
any of the information in this book for yourself, which is your constitutional
right, the author and the publisher assume no responsibility for your actions.

Any people depicted in stock imagery provided by Getty Images are
models, and such images are being used for illustrative purposes only.
Certain stock imagery © Getty Images.

Print information available on the last page.

Scripture taken from the King James Version of the Bible.

THE HOLY BIBLE, NEW INTERNATIONAL VERSION®,
NIV® Copyright © 1973, 1978, 1984, 2011 by Biblica, Inc.®
Used by permission. All rights reserved worldwide.

Scripture taken from the New King James Version®. Copyright ©
1982 by Thomas Nelson. Used by permission. All rights reserved.

ISBN: 978-1-9822-3273-3 (sc)
ISBN: 978-1-9822-3272-6 (hc)
ISBN: 978-1-9822-3274-0 (e)

Library of Congress Control Number: 2019911463

Balboa Press rev. date: 10/21/2019

Contents

Acknowledgments vii
Introduction ix

Chapter 1   Breathe, Smile, and Be at Ease...................... 1
Chapter 2   Listen Attentively to Understand, Not
             to Respond 7
Chapter 3   Resist the Desire to React WAIT
             (Why Am I Talking?
             Why Am I Texting/Tweeting?).......................13
Chapter 4   Give Each Other the Safety to Identify
             and Express Emotions and Feelings............. 25
Chapter 5   Don't Assume; Ask for Clarification.............33
Chapter 6   Don't Take Things Personally.....................43
Chapter 7   Guard against Defensiveness 55
Chapter 8   Relinquish the Need to Be Right.................61
Chapter 9   Be Direct. Be Kind...............................71
Chapter 10   Be Aware of the Power of Your Words......... 79
Chapter 11   Raise Self-Awareness to Guide Reframing... 87
Chapter 12   Shed the Burden of Judgment 95
Chapter 13   Replace Expectations with Hope 103
Chapter 14   Don't Worry. It Doesn't Help....................111
Chapter 15   Let Go of the Need to Control Others........119
Chapter 16   Practice Positive, Compassionate
             Confrontation.................................. 129

Chapter 17 Establish Clear, Healthy Boundaries.......... 141
Chapter 18 Discover the Freedom of Forgiveness 151
Chapter 19 Review, Resolve, and Release Resentments.... 161
Chapter 20 Transform Regret and Remorse 171
Chapter 21 Truth—The Oldest Virtue 179
Chapter 22 Stress Is Inevitable—Use It to Build
            Resilience 187
Chapter 23 Self-Love, Self-Care 195
Chapter 24 Give Only What You Want to Receive 207
Chapter 25 Renew Your Happiness Every Day 213
Chapter 26 Focus on What You Want to Attract—
            Law of Attraction 221
Chapter 27 Redefine Rejection..................................233
Chapter 28 Live in the Present Moment 243
Chapter 29 Be Peaceful 251
Chapter 30 Be Grateful..261
Chapter 31 Bring Back Joy......................................269

Acknowledgments

My heartfelt thanks go to family, including Jamie and Terry, and dear friends who see this as our book, sharing the vision of creating peaceful lives to contribute to a peaceful world. To Eric, Michael, and others who saw my dream evolve, over many years, into this book. To members of our Wednesday group who came early each week to make time to critique all the chapters and offer their encouragement. To John, whose tireless and enthusiastic feedback was priceless. To Nicole, who gave helpful editorial tips, and to Margie for the book cover ideas. To Bill, who was available whenever needed to offer support by exploring the concepts through another pair of eyes, especially in the exciting and stressful last days leading up to submission of the manuscript. To my mother, my first role model for faith and courage. For Divine guidance that showed up in many disguises.

Introduction

When you see yourself changing for the better,
you're creating a better you and a better world.

When questioned regarding the intention of this book, I reflected on input from a client. She saw me as the "tool lady," having spent my life identifying, refining, and practicing the tools that help humans live a peaceful and joyful life. Thus, the word "tool" seemed like a good description of the guidelines offered in the following chapters.

This book is meant to capture the essence of everything I have assimilated and share in groups and individual sessions and with many others. Hopefully, these ideas will be like pebbles thrown into a still lake, spreading out ripples of peace and well-being far and wide.

Change is constant. We cannot remain the same because we are ultimately progressing or regressing through our action or inaction. When we are not growing, we are regressing, like standing still on the down escalator. By taking positive steps, we grow and flourish for the common good and engage in life in a purposeful way.

One of my greatest rewards as a psychotherapist is witnessing others accept guidance, make positive changes, and choose to be grateful, peaceful, and hopeful, moment by moment. This is my hope for you with this book.

Can You See What Eye See is essentially about perception and choices and how these influence growth and peaceful living. Perhaps our most important choice is how we see the world. The optimist looks for the silver lining, whereas the pessimist sees only the dark cloud. The consequence of this choice is hope or despair in the present moment.

There is so much beauty in the world.
You have to develop an eye for beauty to be able to see it.
—*The American Beauty*

I learned my first lesson in the power of perception from my mother. She would often share with me this verse:

Two men looked out from prison bars;
one saw mud, the other stars.
—Frederick Langbridge

My mother's driving force was her faith. Her positive attitude toward life and her innovative approach to challenges were remarkable for a woman of her time. She attributed her accomplishments to her belief that "with God, all things are possible."

To overcome self-made obstacles in writing this book, I needed a helpful definition of success. To me, success would be if it helped one person who was ready to change. This provided the impetus to hit the keys again. When discouraging thoughts arose, I reminded myself that I had to pass on the learning that makes my life peaceful. We are called to be peacemakers.

Can You See What Eye See is a way to share information that was gathered and condensed from the work of inspirational authors, seminars, life experiences, and interactions with fellow travelers along the spiritual path. Quotes highlight these ideas, and teaching stories show how others applied these concepts. These quotes can also be great little pick-me-ups to boost the spirit. Many of these ideas have become ingrained in my thought process, and I have endeavored to research and credit the sources. You may have read or heard some of these insightful, sometimes humorous, messages before, and they will serve as reinforcement. Several participants in the groups I facilitate have come to affectionately refer to these as "Chere-isms."

These tools can be explored on your own as part of your personal journey. The recommendation is to read the chapters sequentially, as they intertwine and overlap. You may also dive into the one that seems more applicable at one time or another. This book will become your toolbox, and you can access the appropriate ones when challenges arise. Over time, you may become comfortable sharing these guidelines with others.

You may also gather like-minded friends to process this book together, or group therapists could use these topics to stimulate discussions, with the benefit of interaction and feedback. Counselors could recommend that their clients read a chapter between sessions to enhance their progress. Anyone can apply these tools to generate healthy and peaceful relationships with themselves and others.

> Life isn't about finding yourself. Life
> is about creating yourself.
> —George Bernard Shaw

Gather your tools and use them in your ongoing process of positive change. Work on becoming an ever-improving version of you. Life is fleeting; let go of suffering and enjoy the journey. One way to be content in uncertainty is to live in the mystery, open, curious, and grateful, and stay in the light.

You will deepen your understanding when you see a situation through the other person's eye. With *Can You See What Eye See*, we will share the vision of peaceful, joyful living and the highest good of all concerned.

CHAPTER 1

Breathe, Smile, and Be at Ease

Love is in the air. Breathe deeply.

Life as we know it begins and ends with the breath. The breath is the most important source of energy. Breathing is normally an involuntary process controlled by the autonomic nervous system without conscious control. Every part of the body needs oxygen to survive. Our bodies work to keep us breathing, even when we are sleeping. It would certainly be tedious if we had to keep track of every breath.

We may take inhaling and exhaling for granted, until the day a common cold restricts our breathing and our most desperate need becomes a simple breath. I think back to a vacation with my sister when I spent two consecutive nights sitting up in bed because I couldn't breathe lying down. Since that time, I have not taken one breath for granted.

In this opening chapter, the breath will also be viewed from the perspective of an effective, voluntary tool; it is the prerequisite for the chapters that follow. Voluntary breathing will be explored in terms of healthy breathing practices and as the first step in handling every challenging situation.

Understanding the power of the breath is like knowing that the brakes in your car are fully functioning before you leave the driveway. You have what it takes to slow down or stop when necessary. When you take a deep breath, you immediately bring about a physiological change, and in stressful interactions, this allows you to shift from an emotional to a logical perspective.

Taking a deep, voluntary breath creates the space for conscious action to avoid impulsive reaction.

This story shows how preoccupation with a situation can disrupt proper breathing. Lia, a client, remarked that during a heated argument, you are not breathing to calm down. You are simply reloading. She revisited an incident of taking rapid breaths on her way to an encounter with her domineering sister. Lia was unaware that shallow breathing meant she was taking in less oxygen and releasing less carbon dioxide, adversely affecting her immune system, mood, and mental clarity. This was raising her physical and emotional stress and could result in dizziness, fainting, nausea, and chest or abdominal pain.

At a stoplight, a police officer looked over at Lia's car. He observed her distressed breathing and asked if she was okay or needed medical assistance. She chuckled nervously, assured him that she was fine, and thanked him for his kind offer. She inhaled, smiled, and returned to the gentle, deep breathing that would release the calming chemicals she needed to restore her composure. Each traffic stop sign gave her the opportunity to stop, breathe, and be alert before proceeding.

Lia had also learned to replace the harmful habit of holding her breath in stressful situations with the healthy alternative of conscious breathing. She understood that when you use proper breathing to stabilize, no one can rob you of your peace.

The breath combined with a smile can be an effective practice. A progressive organization provided an in-service training program on the procedure and benefits of breathing and smiling when taking calls from customers. Then mirrors were installed at the desks of their customer service agents.

This allowed the agents to see how they were coming across to the customers. Within a few months, customer satisfaction improved significantly. and the employees reported feeling more in control and less stressed at the end of their shifts. You could try this experiment yourself the next time you have to make a challenging call.

Ongoing research reveals that breathing correctly keeps the mind and body functioning as it promotes feelings of relaxation, helps you destress, and lowers blood pressure. Slowing your breathing will provide nourishment for body and spirit. For example, scuba divers learn the crucial nature of proper breathing, as do snorkelers when they come up for air. Interestingly, scuba divers are taught to follow the bubbles when needing to know what direction is up in dark water. The breath helps you follow your thoughts when you are in the dark about what to do next.

Studies indicate that deep breaths trigger the parasympathetic nervous system, which helps to calm you. With the awareness that breathing is the essence of life, commit to bringing your full attention to the breath, visualizing how you are energizing and connecting mind, body, and spirit. Witness how the breath can dramatically impact aspects of life, such as anxiety, distressing thoughts, restlessness, and insomnia, and can bring a sense of control over emotions, behaviors, and well-being. Use the breath to get in touch with your inner wisdom and grace. To feel better, breathe better.

> The single most effective relaxation technique
> I know is conscious regulation of breath.
> —Dr. Andrew Weil

This is a simple deep–breathing exercise called belly breathing (a.k.a. diaphragmatic breathing). Lie on your back on a flat surface, bend your knees, and place a cushion under your knees and (or) head for comfort. Rest your hand on your belly to help you concentrate on the air going in and out. Inhale deeply through your nose and feel your stomach rise. Let your belly relax. Breathe out slowly through your pursed lips, like blowing bubbles. Repeat for a few minutes. Increase the time as you become more comfortable with the exercise.

Breathing deeply into your belly will expand your rib cage over time and oxygenate your body more efficiently, which in turn allows your metabolism to become more efficient. When you develop a breathing practice, starting with just five minutes a day at a designated time and sacred space, you train your mind to gently bring you back from overthinking. The breath gives you something concrete to rely on.

Establish and maintain a breathing practice to enhance your mental, physical, and spiritual well-being. The breath becomes your path to health and wellness. Thich Nhat Hanh offers this brief meditation, which is a beneficial daily practice and a great resource in times of stress: "Breathing in I am a mountain. Breathing out I feel solid."

There is a Zen story about a man riding a horse that is galloping frantically. A man standing on the road yells to him, "Where are you going in such a hurry?" The man on the horse yells back, "I don't know. Ask the horse."

Whenever your mind feels like that galloping horse overcome with fear, anxiety, and distractions, the conscious breath can restore your peace of mind. Pay attention to how the breath connects your mind and body. You will regain control, see things more clearly, and proceed effectively.

Life will provide many opportunities for you to behave one way or another. With the awareness that you do not have to react immediately, you use the breath to provide the space to mindfully choose your response. Ted, the father of a precious five-year-old, wanted to prepare her for the potential stress of moving to a new home. He asked her not to worry if Mommy and Daddy got upset at times. His little daughter touched his hand and said, "Daddy, you just need to breathe!" He smiled and hoped she had learned this from him.

> Whenever your mind becomes scattered, use your
> breath as the means to take hold of your mind again.
> —Thich Nhat Hanh

Key Points

- Visualize breathing life into every cell of your body.
- Inhale deeply and exhale slowly through lips.
- Be aware of expanding your rib cage, followed by a gentle release.
- Recognize all the benefits of mindful breathing.
- Practice daily so that this becomes your default mode.
- Access the breath as your first step in handling any situation.
- Be ever grateful for the breath.

The importance of the breath cannot be overstated. Develop your breathing exercises by starting with short time-outs and extend your practice as you become more comfortable. Use the breath as your first and most valuable tool for self-control and inner peace. Take a deep breath and then move on to the other chapters.

CHAPTER 2

Listen Attentively to
Understand, Not to Respond

You cannot truly listen to anyone and do
anything else at the same time.
—Scott Peck

Listening attentively to understand means being fully present and completely focused on what is being said. There is a magnet on my refrigerator that states, "The first rule of love is to listen." This invites you to use the breath to slow down inside, filter out the distractions, and listen quietly with the intention of understanding what is being shared. This reminds you that love is patient and you endeavor to be the compassionate, nonjudgmental observer. It may take a while for the other person to express his or her thoughts and feelings, and you need to refrain from interrupting. Later, there may be the need to clarify what you heard, reinforcing your commitment to listen to understand.

Active listening frees you of the misconception that you have to respond immediately and come up with the solution. You clear out the clutter and calm the mind. Consider a time when a close friend wants to share her challenges, decisions, and fears with you. There is no sense of urgency. She simply needs to explore her thoughts and feelings. She is not asking for a road map to make it through this challenge. You resist the temptation to take over and tell her what you think she should do. If she asks for your input, you verify what you understand and offer feedback for her reflection. Your greatest contribution is to provide the patience and careful consideration to help her unearth the real problem and shift the focus to what really matters. You offer the precious gift of your time and attention.

The deepest expression of Love is paying attention.
—Unknown

The following story is a good example of the above quote.

Manny and Elizabeth had a couple's therapy session during which Manny listened to his wife as she revisited a painful event that he had no memory of because he had been in a blackout after an evening of excessive drinking. He had already made many positive changes in his life and felt he was now ready to give his full attention in order to validate his wife's feelings.

After Elizabeth shared the events of that traumatic night, there was a long silence. Then Manny haltingly said, "I know you are waiting for me to say I am sorry, but I can't do that." Elizabeth shuddered and remained tense and quiet. There was another long silence as Manny collected his thoughts. He continued. "I can't say I am sorry, because that would not even begin to touch all the pain I caused. I regret all the times in the past when I said I was sorry, and then I just repeated the hurtful behaviors. All I can say now is and that I never, ever meant to hurt you, and I will do everything in my power to be the husband you deserve. It is time for me to express my apology through my actions, not my words. I hope to be worthy of your forgiveness." Elizabeth exhaled, as if releasing the tension from her body. He gently touched her hand, and she gave a little nod.

It would have been very easy to misinterpret Manny's

first words and the heavy silence that followed. The ability to patiently sit in that discomfort made a vital difference in the outcome of the conversation. They vowed to always make time to truly listen.

> The word "listen" contains the same
> letters as the word "silent."
> —Alfred Brendel

When was the last time you felt really heard? What was that experience like? What would it be like for you to give this attention to the other person? *Mindfulness for Beginners* describes deep listening as the essence of mindfulness. How many times in the past have you had to go back over a conversation to be able to unravel all the misunderstandings, realizing that what you thought you heard someone say was not what they meant?

A hypothesis first advanced by Edward Sapir in 1929 and subsequently developed by his student Benjamin Whorf suggested that an individual's thoughts and actions are greatly influenced by the language or languages that individual speaks, characteristic of the culture in which it is spoken. This became known as the Sapir Whorf hypothesis. Although this has drawn some disagreement in the linguistic arena, it does highlight the value of listening, clarifying, and understanding in relationships.

Today, people of different regions and cultures find themselves in a melting pot through travel, immigration, and scholastic endeavors. Relating to the thinking and actions of the girl next door in a small town where you grew up may seem simple compared to the complexity of trying to coexist with someone from across the world with differences in native language and culture. Perhaps instead of working so hard to be interesting, endeavor to be interested. Many guides have messages for you when you listen with an open mind, free of opinions and judgment.

Listening, including listening to yourself, requires the essential ingredient of patience. Think of a time when you had a gut feeling and you took the time to explore the feeling. You were probably unaware that your gut feelings about a person or a situation have a neurological basis. Scientists have determined that the neurons that line the stomach are filled with chemicals called neurotransmitters, which facilitate communication among nerve cells. One key neurotransmitter is serotonin, which plays a role in emotional regulation that is not fully understood. Scientists have also discovered that while serotonin is found in the brain, around 90 percent of the body's supply is in the gut. This indicates that your body has two brains, the one in the skull and the less well-known and very valuable one in the human gut. They have been compared to Siamese twins; when one experiences a feeling, so does the other. The ability to slow down, listen, and interpret gut feelings can greatly enhance decision-making, keeping you safe and peaceful.

From a physical perspective, another interesting piece of research reveals that having enough healthy bacteria in the gut has the potential to impact the communication between the brain and the gut and thus regulate mood. It goes on to suggest that beneficial bacteria in the gut will increase GABA receptors in the brain to alleviate mood disorders like chronic depression. With this in mind, you might consider adding probiotics such as *Lactobacillus* and *Bifidobacterium* to your supplements to increase the healthy bacteria in your system and enhance positive feelings. As with all supplements, you would need to seek medical advice in the event of any contraindications based on your health status or current medication.

The Navajo had a special way of speaking: they spoke

and then had silence. They believed the silence was more informative than the word, and unless we allowed silence, we would never have the full meaning of what the words were.

I define connection as the energy that exists between people when they feel seen, heard, and valued; when they can give and receive without judgment; and when they derive sustenance and strength from the relationship.
—Brené Brown

Key Points

- Breathe.
- Clear out any distractions.
- Be patient.
- Don't interrupt.
- Let go of the need to provide the solution.
- Focus on understanding what is being said.
- Give physical indications that you are attentive: nods, eye contact, appropriate touch, and so on.
- Give feedback if asked. Begin by clarifying what you heard.

You have the opportunity to deepen your connection with your loved ones. Your greatest gift is your undivided attention. Incorporating these ideas of patience, curiosity, presence, nonjudgment, and openness, free of the need to provide a solution, can be challenging in this fast-paced world. This will be a wise investment of that valuable commodity: your time. You may discover that you actually save time and feel more peaceful and loving.

CHAPTER 3

Resist the Desire to React WAIT (Why Am I Talking? Why Am I Texting/Tweeting?)

Reactive people are everywhere—in traffic and shopping centers, on forums and social networks, on television and in the news, at work, everywhere. How can you avoid being seduced into reacting in anger or other emotions?

Acronyms like WAIT are sprinkled throughout this book to help you, at the right moment, access the tool you need. When you choose to apply WAIT, *Why am I talking?* can be closely followed by *What am I thinking?*

> Words empty as the wind are best left unsaid.
> —Homer

WAIT works in tandem with the pause button, like a two-person kayak. The concept of the pause button provides an image, along with a physical action, to interrupt the progression of reacting impulsively. You can stop right now and install your own pause button, choosing a spot like your wrist or knee. Taking a deep conscious breath, as suggested in chapter 1—or better still, taking three conscious breaths to lower the intensity—and hitting your pause button gives you time to think it through more clearly and dispassionately.

Visualize how your pause button could put everything on hold, allowing you to become a detached witness.

> Self-control is our greatest strength.
> —Roy Baumeister

The intention is to move from reactive to responsive, having your thoughts and actions move from fear to love. Applying your pause button provides the important space between the event and your response to the event. In the moments of silence, both the speaker and listener can reflect on what was said and what each person felt.

Think of a situation when words were tossed mindlessly back and forth, becoming increasing hurtful, and in retrospect, it all seemed so pointless. When you WAIT, you take full responsibility, and you no longer have to justify your reactive behaviors by blaming someone else.

> Between stimulus and response there is a space. In that space is our power to choose our response. In our response lie our growth and our freedom.
> —Viktor E. Frankl

There are some words that are your trigger words, because they have a specific meaning for you. They can disrupt the communication by taking your thoughts in a completely different direction. When this happens, you miss the rest of the conversation and react to the intensity of the meaning of the word or words for you. Feelings from old unresolved issues surface, and the intensity of your reaction seems out of proportion to the current event. As Star Trek first officer, Spock, said to Captain Kirk, "Insults are effective only where emotion is present."

Can You See What Eye See?

This story illustrates the need to WAIT and honor thoughts and feelings. Janet was sorting the mail and stopped to leaf through a magazine from a local college. She said pensively to her husband, Bob, "I wonder if I would enjoy going back to college and finishing my degree at this late stage." Bob's immediate reply was "Well, that sounds like a silly waste of time to me." Janet dropped the magazine and left the room in tears.

Janet had to figure out what had caused such intense feelings. She surrendered to the feelings, hoping to make the connection to the first time she had felt like that. This gradually opened an old wound for Janet. She recalled an event when she was about ten years old. She and her austere father, a physician whose love and validation she had always longed for, were in the attic sorting through collectibles. She picked up an old stethoscope and said wistfully, "Maybe I'll be doctor like you or a nurse." Her father exploded and said, "Oh for heaven's sake, being a nurse is like being a glorified maid, and women are too silly to be doctors." Janet, a quiet, introverted little girl, was deeply hurt. She hid her silent tears and buried that old, painful memory. When Bob used that word "silly," a wave of old feelings overwhelmed her. She heard her father's cold, condescending tone, and all her buried pain and insecurities came flooding back.

Had Janet automatically reacted, an exchange of angry words could have escalated into a fight with Bob. She recalled Dr. Weisinger's time-out technique, modified from the original version where a disruptive child would be removed from a situation (classroom, dinner table, etc.) for a designated period. In this version, you remove yourself to reappraise the situation. You say, "I am beginning to feel angry, and I want to take a time-out." Then you take it. Having the time and space to access her old, repressed feelings, she was able to identify and defuse the power of that trigger. Having gained insight, she could work on resolving the issue.

As you give your attention and compassion to your actions and reactions, you get more in touch with your inner self, and growth is an ongoing process. You learn that you are reacting to a perceived attack, and you can change your perception and guard your peace.

In this example, Greta also had the opportunity to use WAIT on her first business trip to another city. She had mustered up her courage to be able to handle her presentation with grace and professionalism. In all her preparation, she had not factored in the possibility of a flat tire with her rental car. She pulled over to the side of the expressway. All decked out in her suit and high heels, she stared at the tire while she gathered her thoughts.

She was a little startled as a truck approached and pulled over, and a rather grizzly-looking man lumbered over. He took one look at her and the flat tire and said, "I don't know what you're waiting for. Must be 'cause you're one of them city women or you're pretty ignorant, to be looking so pitiful." She inhaled, fighting off the threatening tears. The stranger shrugged, and Greta was surprised when he did a chivalrous act. He changed her tire. With a wave, he was off with his parting remark. "That's the kind of dumb problem my daughter would get into."

She was not sure he heard her thanking him as he walked toward his truck. She took some breaths and reflected on how grateful she was for his unsolicited help and that she had not reacted to his brash remarks. After all, she was a woman who lived in the city, ignorant of many things, and—who knows—perhaps she had been looking a little pitiful. There was no point in taking offense. She needed her energy to pull herself together and proceed to her presentation. She chuckled as she drove away, thinking that this odd man had been her knight in "rusty armor."

Can You See What Eye See?

Your perception of me is a reflection of you;
my reaction to you is an awareness of me.

—Unknown

Here is another suggestion for the times when a person says something to you that seems antagonistic. Your knee-jerk reaction would be to engage in the escalating hostility. Using your recently installed pause button, softly and slowly say, "WOW!" (Wait, observe, wonder.) This immediately releases tension, like letting a little steam out of the top of a pressure cooker. This breaks the progression of angry retorts and gives you time to breathe and think about if and how you choose to respond. You can ponder what would cause the other person to be so combative.

Often the excuse for reacting is "He pushed my buttons," which then attempts to place blame on the other person. When you realize that these are your buttons, you can disconnect these buttons, replace them with your pause button, and refrain from reacting in ways that you later regret. In any research project, the mouse will continue to push the lever as long as there is some type of reward. Reacting to a perceived attack may reinforce the unwanted behaviors.

Nothing gives one person so much advantage over another
as to remain cool and unruffled under all circumstances.
—Thomas Jefferson

Think about fishing. The fisherman throws out his line, and the fish that takes the bait may get caught. Become the smart fish that learns how to observe the lure and not get hooked. You can develop the inner strength to refrain from an immediate reaction as you calmly consider your options. You keep in mind that your words define you. You can commit to remain as master of your own emotions and take responsibility for every word that leaves your lips.

Those who remain tranquil, when they perceive another's anger, protect themselves and all other beings.
—The Tibetan Dhammapada

Unexpected shifts in your emotional state can occur. Without warning, you could feel overwhelmed, accompanied by physical manifestations such as a racing heart, shortness of breath, or difficulty breathing. You strive to identify the source. You reflect on conversations with a particular friend who makes snide little digs (Spanish *pullitas*). You thought you had been disregarding them. You get in touch with how these remarks have been impacting you internally. You realize that you have been absorbing and stacking these provoking remarks. You were repressing the feelings (an unconscious action) until you reached your limit. Experiencing distress was your body's wake-up call to alert you to take corrective action.

You learn how to clear out the pile of stress with conscious effort. You revisit past conversations and validate each feeling you experienced at the time. You give your full attention to the feelings until they diminish, and you can acknowledge that this person's behavior has been disrupting your peace. When similar situations occur, you may choose to suppress your feelings (a conscious action) as a temporary coping skill for self-control, and you return to process and release them later. Changing your perception of the behaviors is another effective technique (chapter 11, "Reframing"). Depending on the depth of your friendship, you may invite your friend to process this with you to gain a better understanding and change the dynamic. This may have to be revisited from time to time, as one or the other falls back into the old pattern. You might decide to limit your conversations with this person, especially on hot topics.

This event shows the value of refraining from retaliation. Billy had just purchased his new car, a Firebird. He loved everything about it and wanted to show it off to his girlfriend. He asked her to meet him at his mother's condo for a surprise. He parked on the side near the entrance of the walkway, thinking he would just be a couple of minutes. His girlfriend and his mother were deep in conversation, and he waited anxiously to have them both come to see his new car.

It took longer than expected, and when they got outside, there was a violation sticker on the window on the driver's side of his brand new car. Feeling a little irritated, he decided to peel it off. He discovered that it had been affixed with very strong glue, not just on the corners but on every inch of the paper, and the sun had baked in into the window. In his attempts to remove the sticker with a scraper, he scratched the glass.

Billy felt a rush of anger at the malice of the guard and the unnecessary damage to the window. He asked his mother if she had a can of spray paint. His mother said she did but wondered why he needed this. Billy explained that he was so angry at the vindictive action of the guard that he was going to spray-paint the door to the management office. His mother said to Billy, "You are really angry at his behavior, so take a moment to think about this. If you damage property, how will your behavior be any different from his?" Billy stopped in his tracks. He knew his mother was right. She had taught him all his life not to allow another person's spitefulness to influence his behavior. Her guidance activated his self-regulation. He took a deep breath and thanked his mother for her wisdom.

> Don't do something permanently stupid just
> because you're temporarily upset.
> —Author unknown

Reacting is closely aligned to seeking revenge. Once you are seduced into seeking revenge for a perceived injustice, your behavior is essentially no different from the behavior of the perpetrator, and evil wins again. Revenge feeds on itself. You move from being the victim to being the villain and thereby earn the consequences of your behavior, whatever your philosophy might be—the universal law of karma, cause and effect, do unto others as you would have others do unto you, what I give to you I give to myself. It all comes back to trusting that there is a power greater than you who is handling the details. When you react in fear, you give away your power and become a part of the collective fear.

> Not acting in anger when you are angry
> requires the intention of love.
> —Gary Zukav

Stop, look, listen, feel. In challenging moments, you can strengthen your self-control with the traffic light formula. Picture a traffic light. The red light at the top bids you, "Stop!" This image will alert you that reacting impulsively without conscious thought is dangerous. Take that deep, calming breath. This is the time to hit the emotional brakes. Moving down to the amber light, this is the time to *look* and *listen*. Go to curiosity and observe the event from different perspectives. By giving your full attention, you slow down and feel empowered. Finally, you go down to the green light, where you *feel* calm enough to be able to determine what is the next best course of action or inaction. The image of a traffic light can be a good reminder.

> You who know better, must do better.
> —Jamaican proverb

Another handy technique to use when someone asks you a question or gives advice in a harsh, abrasive tone is to take the time to separate the words from the tone. If the question or advice is in any way helpful, you can take the words and pass them through your "transformer" to hear the words as if they had been said in a respectful, effective manner. Rather than be triggered to react poorly or be aggravated, you can respond to your improved version of the words, keeping what is beneficial and disregarding the rest. Sometimes good advice is rejected because of the irritating presentation. Neil shared that when it all becomes too stressful and chaotic, he thinks about Diana Ross and the Supremes extending their palms and singing, "Stop—in the name of love." Then it is not possible to take things too seriously.

> Love is my gift to the world. I fill myself with love
> and send that love out into the world. How others
> treat me is their path; how I react is mine.
> —Dr. Wayne Dyer

When I saw the movie *Love Story* years ago, I could not make sense of that famous line from the movie, "Love means never having to say I'm sorry." However, years later, my interpretation was, "Love means never saying anything unkind that I will need to go back later and say I'm sorry about." A lofty goal indeed! Must admit the phrase is not as catchy.

Jimmy's story shows how practicing restraint can bring a new feeling of empowerment. He and his wife had another disagreement. Their old pattern was that the next morning, each would apologize: "I'm sorry," followed by "You know I didn't mean it" (excuse), "You made me mad" (blame), "You said it first" (justification), "You always hurt me" (victim), and "Oh just get over it" (egoist). This time, he applied his new tools, and the outcome was different. Having not said anything belligerent, Jimmy didn't need to apologize. He hoped that his wife would notice and be motivated to take similar steps to foster inner peace and a loving relationship.

Awareness is equally important if you are the person who delays reacting or responding indefinitely. You take too long deliberating on the issue and the end result is avoidance rather than resolution. You dread another difficult conversation. It seems easier to dismiss the issue, thinking it will go away, but the tension builds up and is detrimental to your well-being and your relationship. Make the conscious effort to learn healthy ways to process the event, increase understanding of the underlying message, and move forward peacefully (chapter 16).

This final Zen story illustrates the anger within. A monk wants to meditate by himself. He takes his boat out to the middle of the lake, moors it there, closes his eyes, and begins his meditation. After a few hours of undisturbed silence, he suddenly feels the bump of another boat colliding with his own. With his eyes still closed, he senses his anger rising, and by the time he opens his eyes, he is ready to scream at the boatman who dared to disturb his meditation. But when he opens his eyes, he sees it's an empty boat that probably got untethered and floated to the middle of the lake. At that moment, the monk achieves self-realization and understands that the anger is within him; it merely needs the bump of an external object to provoke it out of him. From then on, whenever he comes across someone who irritates him or provokes him to anger, he reminds himself, "The other person is merely an empty boat. The anger is within me."

You can apply this learning in your own life. When the actions of others provoke you, you are reminded that you have more work to do to find healthy ways to free yourself of the anger within.

The most important thing we learned is that self-control—and the ability to regulate one's own emotions—involves a set of skills that can be taught and learned. They're acquirable.
—Walter Mischel

Key Points

- Breathe.
- Hit your pause button.
- WAIT—why am I talking before I understand what am I thinking?
- Use the WOW tool to release tension (wait, observe, wonder).
- Identify your feelings and clarify what you understood.
- Use the traffic light technique: stop, look, listen, feel.
- Determine if a response is necessary—now, later, or ever.
- Validate your effort to remain calm and peaceful.

How might your life experience be altered by installing your own pause button and learning to WAIT? Anger is a complex emotion, and as with other emotions—sadness, joy, loneliness, and so on—you can validate your anger and determine healthy ways to express and transform it. See yourself as the agent of peace through self-mastery, rather than as a reflection of chaos. Self-restraint is a measure of your strength. When you are aware that something or someone has activated negative feelings, you can consciously claim your peace and feel the positive energy return to you. You take back your power when you STOP: stop, take a breath, observe, proceed peacefully.

CHAPTER 4

Give Each Other the Safety to Identify and Express Emotions and Feelings

People feel really most alive when they are able
to express who they are and how they feel.
—Mihaly Csikszentmihalyi

Think of a relationship where each gives the other the freedom to think aloud, secure in the knowledge that it will be safe to be open and unguarded, free of the fear of being judged or ridiculed. What would be involved in making this type of commitment? A good starting place would be self-exploration and an understanding of the role of emotions and feelings.

A brief explanation from current research is emotions are physical and instinctual, the fight-or-flight response, involving a release of chemicals throughout the brain and body. Feelings are set off by emotions within seconds, influenced by personal beliefs, experiences, and memories.

With the realization that emotions can hijack the brain, conscious effort can help to clarify and regulate thoughts and behaviors. You can take the time to explore each situation and process your own unique reaction.

When asked if everything is okay, rather than hide your feelings, you can be open. It may seem easier to suppress, dismiss, or ignore the feelings, until you recognize that these are temporary coping methods that do not bring understanding or peace in the long term. Feelings are not facts, and you need to reflect on how your perception of reality influences your feelings.

When you have established a relationship in which you can share freely, you can have the benefit of another pair of ears to help you separate facts, emotions, and feelings. You can relax and reflect on the feedback you have invited and be equally considerate when the roles are reversed. You validate and reaffirm the comfort of being able to share freely with a trusted partner. This is the precious gift you can offer each other, based on a common goal of deepening the trust and intimacy in the relationship.

> Mankind are governed more by their
> feelings than by reason.
> —Samuel Adams

Robert's story shows how he learned to improve his relationship with his son. His son was becoming more and more distant to the point of limiting his responses to "Yes," "No," or "I don't know," whenever possible. As each was invited to explore what was happening, it became evident that his son did not feel safe to express any thoughts and feelings to Robert for fear of the angry, sometimes volatile, reactions.

Robert listened quietly and then took full responsibility for his erratic retorts in many conversations. He was able to come to terms with his estranged relationship with his own father. Sadly, he was becoming everything he hated about his father.

Thus, the process of change began. Robert made the decision to revisit his own painful childhood with his abusive father. At age sixteen, Robert had found the courage to stand up to his father and tell him that he would no longer be allowed to continue to treat him, his mother, and his siblings aggressively. His father bristled with rage and abruptly fled from the room. His father retreated into silence and never spoke to Robert again. Robert had always longed for his father's validation. After this confrontation, his father's rageful outbursts were replaced with cold indifference. Robert became aware of how this old pain returned whenever his son's way of coping with their stressful relationship was to retreat into silence. As Robert came to terms with the whole dynamic, understanding led to change and opened the path to healing. Robert followed through on the initial recommendation. He made the commitment to his son that going forward he would create a safe space for his son to express thoughts and feelings, and that if at any time he caught himself falling back into old, harsh behaviors, he would stop immediately and apologize.

His son cautiously agreed to take the risk of being more open with his father. Robert was invited to give his son a special word to say to him whenever his son sensed that the conversation was heading in the wrong direction. This would provide another safeguard for Robert. Robert chose the word "regroup," and his son agreed to say this word to Robert to interrupt the escalation of anger.

This brought Robert hope that he could take action to heal the anguish with his own father as well as change his hurtful behaviors that had caused the distance in his relationship with his son. Robert saw he could have the loving relationship that he and his son had believed was impossible. Now they knew they could build a new track record and develop trust.

Subsequent sessions guided them to improve their communication. They were invited to keep the focus on the relationship they hoped to build and to bear this in mind before they said or did anything, by asking themselves this question: "Will this take me closer or farther away from the relationship I want to build?" They learned to validate the things they agreed on, knowing that there would be times when they could disagree without being disrespectful of the other's opinion.

> Educating the mind without educating
> the heart is no education at all.
> —Aristotle

There was Vince's story. Prompted by the realization that his marriage was falling apart, Vince made the decision to seek help. He said his wife would often accuse him of having no feelings—and certainly having no regard for hers. Vince was so out of touch with his own feelings that his first therapy assignment was to read a list of feelings and try to identify any that resonated with him. Next, he learned that every thought matters, and in order to change his feelings, he would need to change his thoughts.

He found the courage to revisit his childhood and recalled the family dynamic of a father who spoke openly about his irritation of overworking to support a family of "parasites." His mother, who lived in this stark, loveless marriage, was often overwhelmed by her three sons. She would compile a list of all their misbehaviors to present to their father to apply the punishment, which was often excessive. Their family code was "Don't talk, don't trust, don't feel," reflective of their dysfunctional family.

One day, Vince haltingly told his mother that his school bus driver had fondled him inappropriately. He had longed for the safety of sharing this dark secret with his mother and feeling the comfort of her compassion. She listened in stony silence. Later that evening, during one of their fierce arguments, his mother shouted this information to his father. She immediately regretted doing this when she saw the look of rage on his face. His father stormed out, and the following day, he dragged the driver off the bus and beat him so badly he had to be hospitalized. After this violent incident, the people in their small town avoided Vince. Instead of receiving the social support he needed, he felt even more victimized and alone.

His feelings shut down. He vowed that he would never trust anyone again, and he buried this experience. He excelled in computer science and became a high-powered executive with his company. He married Gracie, a woman he admired, and she believed her love would change him and make him feel more comfortable in social settings. When the years went by and Vince sank deeper into his isolation, Gracie felt unloved and turned to alcohol, and their unhappiness increased. Realizing that he was losing the only kind person in his life, he agreed to seek professional help. He had seldom thought of the childhood incident and had never spoken of it again until that moment in therapy.

When Vince identified what was driving his pain, he was encouraged by the prospect of changing his life. He also became aware that whenever Gracie would point out any inappropriate behavior, he would react by inflicting the kind of hurtful remark he had witnessed throughout his parents' marriage. He would feel immediately ashamed when he would see Gracie's silent tears. They knew they had to stop the pain.

They realized that their love could only flourish in a safe place. Vince and Gracie learned how to listen and validate each other as each took the risk of exploring reactions and feelings. They were guided to let go of fear and grow in the same direction, having the comfort of being open and receptive.

They were also invited to incorporate an "affection check-in" practice, where no words were spoken. Each would take a moment to breathe and get close to experience a heart-to-heart communication, allowing their hearts to touch and speak to each other. This would be a nonverbal expression of simultaneous giving and receiving, creating the synergy of energy to generate more love and connection. Vince had come from a family that did not show affection, and he felt uncomfortable about doing the exercise. He looked at Gracie and could see that she wanted to take this step. He reluctantly agreed. The practice was adapted to start off with closing their eyes and holding hands until Vince relaxed and felt more comfortable. He was rewarded for his willingness. The affection check-in exercise became a brief time-out from thinking and all the distractions of their busy lives, to affirm their love.

> Trust is believing I will be safe with you.
> Love is striving to keep that trust.
> —Wordlions

Challenging situations can also arise when you do not know how to be supportive. For example, when a friend is facing a loss or potential loss of a loved one due to adverse events, such as a life-threatening accident or a fatal illness, you might wonder what is the right thing to say or do. You come to understand that you don't have to say anything. You can be a listener if the person wants to talk, or you can sit in comfortable silence, simply offering to be there if needed. You provide a safe sounding board.

When Jackie's daughter had a seizure and had to be placed in a medically induced coma, her friends and family felt inadequate to help her through the fear of uncertainty. What she really needed was someone to listen as all her pent-up feelings exploded: from anger, to sadness, to self-pity, to sorrow, and back to pain and anger. She did not want to hear that she shouldn't be angry with God, or that they understood how she was feeling, or for them to share traumatic events from their past. She wanted to be able to unburden all the feelings that were swirling around in her brain until she could become exhausted and find her way back to sanity and peace.

This was a time when Jackie needed a safe place to explore and express feelings, to be able to honor her distress until she was able to reconnect with the "faith that surpasses understanding." For Jackie's family and friends, this was an opportunity to accept their own discomfort and be consciously present and compassionate, providing the safe place that she needed.

> Being a good friend doesn't mean you always have
> to have the right words to say. Sometimes is means
> you just have to know when to be a good listener.
> —Katrina Meyer

For the person who grew up in an environment where feelings were never shared or feelings were invalidated, the response to the question "How are you?" is automatically "Fine!" The goal becomes to create that safe space in your relationship by giving each other the assurance that anything can be explored calmly without fear of hurtful reactions or unsolicited advice. You remain vigilant in recognizing and correcting any early signs of reverting to old thinking. Feeling safe contributes greatly to the emotional connection that the heart needs. When you strive to create safety in your relationships, the benefits of human connection are immeasurable.

> At the end of the day, the goals are
> simple: safety and security.
> —Jodi Rell

Key Points

- Breathe.
- Give your loved ones the safety to express thoughts and feelings.
- Put yourself in the other person's place.
- Practice patience to build trust.
- Be gentle.
- Be a compassionate listener.

Building blocks for creating safety are think, feel, filter, speak. Each interaction is an opportunity to show that you can be vulnerable with each other and deepen understanding. Earning trust over time will reinforce the commitment to share thoughts and feelings safely, including validating the positive. This process will extend to the others in your life, especially your children, who absorb everything they experience in the space between their two role models. This is where they witness their first important lessons for life's journey.

CHAPTER 5

Don't Assume; Ask for Clarification

The problem with making assumptions is
that we believe they are the truth.
—Anonymous

You may be old enough to remember the show *Dragnet* where
Sergeant Friday would interrupt the victim's or witness's
lengthy report with his famous words, "Just the facts,
ma'am." Yet, is it possible to give just the facts? How does
the past with its wealth of experiences and social influence
affect our perception of the present?

Much has been written about the subconscious. An
effective analogy is to picture entering a large, dark room.
Switch on a flashlight. The small area that is illuminated by
the light represents the conscious, and all the rest of the dark
room is the unconscious. With this image in mind, you get
some understanding of the extensiveness of the subconscious
as a reservoir of past events, especially unresolved issues.

The way you think determines the way you feel,
and the way you feel influences the way you act.
—Rick Warren and Craig Sager (adapted)

Beliefs often fuel assumptions. Events in our lives
are processed through a series of filters. Dr. Albert Ellis

developed the ABC model to explain the connection among (A) activating event / adversity, (B) our beliefs, and (C) the consequence / your thoughts and feelings. Thus, you discover the power of your belief system and how this translates an event into thoughts, and these thoughts transfer into feelings that influence your behavior. When you acknowledge the feeling, you can identify the belief that is creating this response and, if necessary, challenge whether the belief is true. It is important to understand how our perception shapes our reality.

> Your opinion is your opinion. Your perception is your perception. Do not confuse them with "facts" or "truths."
> —John Moore

One of the most common assumptions is that others think, feel, and act the way we do. When the other does not respond the way we assumed he or she would, we make up a story to explain the behavior and justify our distress.

This story shows how assumptions can be a setup for disappointment. Ana went on vacation with friends shortly after she started dating Robert. This was before the cell phone era, and making a long distance call took more effort. The first night of her trip, she called Robert, assuming that he would respond with the same enthusiasm that she would have portrayed had the situation been reversed. When Robert answered the phone, he was in the middle of a card game with his son and other friends, so he spoke briefly, thanked her for the call, and then they hung up. Ana felt disappointed at his casual response. She immediately began creating the story that he obviously did not care the way she did, and she regretted having made the call in the first place.

As their relationship developed, Ana learned that she and Robert responded quite differently to events; whereas she was more demonstrative and outgoing, Robert was more even-tempered and reserved. Over time, they deepened their understanding. Ana came to accept that Robert expressed his feelings more subtly, and Robert endeavored to be more open in sharing his thoughts and feelings. Through clarification, they were able to move closer rather than have their differences create distance in their relationship.

Assumptions can be even more misleading when you do not have all the information, and you spin your own story until it becomes a full-length movie. This movie is seldom positive and brings a range of negative, distressing feelings. The more attention you give to your movie, the more unnecessary discomfort you will experience. Thus, you suffer in advance for something that may or may not have any basis in reality.

> The hardest assumption to challenge is the one
> you don't even know you are making.
> —Douglas Adams

Consider the situation with Tom and Mary and the role of assumptions in projecting feelings. Tom is in a treatment program, and he has invited Mary, his wife, to attend the weekly family group. Tom has a history of abandonment issues, an absentee father who was never able to come to Tom's school events, not even to his graduation from college. Mary was the daughter of an alcoholic father. She grew up watching her mother take on more and more responsibility. Her mother never made time for herself and felt unappreciated and overwhelmed most of the time.

Tom had arrived early for group and had been anxiously glancing back and forth until he saw Mary enter the room. Mary rushed in just as the group was about to start. She slipped in quietly beside Tom. She sighed. Impacted by their assumptions, these facts are interpreted and experienced accordingly.

His story was that Mary probably didn't really want to be there (just like his father, who never showed up for anything important in his life), and that was evident by her sigh. Obviously his group was not important to her, and in fact maybe she didn't even care about his recovery. He resorted to his old belief that he could not rely on anyone, so why should he expect support from his wife? Perhaps she didn't want to be there, and this was an imposition. His negative self-talk confirmed that he was worthless because he had disappointed her so many times. His conclusion was that he was really alone, and he would never ask her to do anything for him again. His behavior was to ignore her and crawl back into his shell.

Mary, on the other hand, saw Tom's tense facial expression as she entered the room, as if he were scolding her for not arriving earlier. Her story was that, here again, she had not done enough. Nothing she did for anyone was ever enough (just like her demanding, needy family). She felt that this was really unreasonable of Tom, especially since she had had such a stressful day. It had been really hard to get out of the office, fight the traffic, and arrive before the group started. Clearly, she would never measure up to Tom's expectations. He probably thought she was not a supportive wife, and he may not even love her. Her conclusion was she would have to try even harder to please him and still take care of all the other tasks. She suppressed the resentment building in her chest. With a sigh, she shrugged her shoulders and sat despondently in her chair.

Only later when Tom and Mary had the opportunity to revisit and process the event was each of them able to see how reality had been distorted by the story each had created. They realized how often throughout their relationship they had created stories that were full of assumptions about each other's feelings and behavior. They knew they had to break this pattern. They made the commitment to work on their communication and recognize when they were falling back into assuming. With this awareness, they would make the shift to seeking clarification for better understanding to strengthen their relationship.

Assumptions are the termites of relationships.
—Henry Winkler

In day to day interchanges, seeking clarity and providing feedback set the stage for better understanding. You check in with each other to determine if what you are thinking is accurate. You achieve mutual understanding of the dynamic. You are able to identify and share what you learned and how you can apply this to improve future interactions. You are motivated to change because you recall the times that you were immersed in confusing dialogue and hurt feelings, and later had to review and unravel a series of misunderstandings. Applying the brakes at the first sign that the conversation is being derailed to clarify thoughts and feelings, will avoid unnecessary pain and wasted time.

To enhance the communication process, you need to ask clear and direct questions to generate clear and direct answers. You can simplify the exchange by asking one question at a time, rather than imparting a string of questions and comments. "Can you pick Susie up at two o'clock, and if so, can you call the school to let them know? Or, otherwise, could you check with Bobbie to see if she's doing car pool today—unless you can't, in which case I will just have to do it, and that's really going to be almost impossible because of my mandatory meetings." Whew! By the end of the monologue, the recipient has become lost in the barrage of options and has forgotten the original question.

An interesting suggestion to alleviate this type of miscommunication is to work together to create a no-nag list. Display the list in a prominent place, for example the refrigerator. All the tasks are written there, and each person commits to handle specific tasks and include a date of completion. This removes the need for constant reminders that are prompted by the worry that someone might forget the assignment. If there is a valid reason to extend the due date, the person who is responsible for this task makes a written notation of the new target date. This puts all the responsibility on the individual and eliminates the need to nag. A sense of satisfaction is experienced as each person places a check mark beside each task upon completion. This can transform resistance into cooperation and provide an opportunity to express gratitude. This practice has often carried over into creating a personal list and enjoying the feeling of accomplishment. This has also served to reduce procrastination.

Bernice's story illustrates how assumptions distorted crucial events in her life. During her childhood, she had seen her father as this fun, easygoing parent and her mother as this workaholic, cold person who never had any time for her. She decided that she would be very different in her own marriage. She met and fell in love with Daniel, and she knew that her love would make the marriage work. When Daniel turned out to be emotionally unavailable, she worked even harder to make him love her in the way she wanted. They never discussed what each wanted from the relationship. Over the years, she became disillusioned.

Bernice gained a more realistic view of her parents' relationship. Her "workaholic" mother had to have two jobs because her "easygoing" father could never hold a job. A very likeable, charming man, he was unable to be a supportive partner to her mother. What Bernice had assumed was her mother's cold personality, in reality, was the result of exhaustion from being the breadwinner and the homemaker who ran the home, disciplined and guided the children, and lived a selfless life.

She decided to seek clarity in her relationships, especially her marriage. She learned to question what she was thinking and feeling and take the time to explore with the other person what he or she meant. Improving communication led the way to breaking the old habit of reacting to assumptions.

One of the most devastating assumptions was when Romeo found Juliet, who had been drugged, and, assuming that she was dead, took his own life.

It is quite easy to fall under the spell of assumptions.
—Steven Redhead, *Life Is Simply a Game*

Think of the times when someone may have said to you, "I know exactly what you are feeling right now," or "I know you better than you know yourself." These words can immediately create distance and curtail further communication. Thoughts and feelings are constantly changing, so it is unrealistic to assume that you know what another person is thinking or feeling. As you grow and evolve, you learn that beliefs can exist at a subconscious level, and you challenge your own chronic perceptions.

People may listen to a presenter give an unbiased lecture by exploring both sides of the topic, yet each person is more likely to see and hear the version that supports their belief. Preconceived opinions can influence the way your mind processes communication.

What your eyes see, what your ears hear
is often what is already in your mind.
—Unknown

A speaker told this cute story at a workshop. He overheard his eight-year-old son at a family gathering say to his cousin, "God is dead." Being a little alarmed to hear this, he decided to bring this up later. The next day, he shared with his son that he had overheard him telling his cousin that God was dead, and he wondered what that was about. His son replied simply, "Well, Daddy, Grandpa Lee is in heaven, and he is dead. God is in heaven, so he must be dead too." What a relief to discover that his eight-year-old son was not quoting Nietzsche! Asking for clarification revealed that there was a reasonable explanation.

By exploring, rather than assuming, the father avoided a lot of confusion. It is similar to having your child ask where babies come from, and before you take off on an hour-long, complex biological explanation, you pause and get some clarity, only to discover that the question was asked to determine, "Will Mommy get my new baby brother at the hospital?"

The way to keep yourself from making
assumptions is to ask questions.
—Don Miguel Ruiz

If you should observe that your friend is tearful, rather than assuming sadness, you may ask, "I see your tears. How are you feeling?" Who knows? This could be the result of allergies! The gift of your awareness can foster sharing and processing of information.

Key Points

- Breathe.
- Observe what you see and what you hear.
- Clarify your understanding.
- Ask questions to invite other perspectives.
- Be open and receptive to new information.

It is time to break your crystal ball and cancel your subscription to *Mind Reading 101*! When you are tempted to assume how someone is feeling, replace your assumption with curiosity. Curiosity, not assumptions, opens a path to understanding. Conversations can become so much simpler and more respectful and meaningful.

Chapter 6

Don't Take Things Personally

What other people think of me is none of my business.
One of the highest places you can get to is being
independent of the good opinions of other people.
—Dr. Wayne Dyer

Several authors have invited us to avoid taking things personally. People often ask, "How can you not takes things personally if something is said directly about you? What if someone said you were plain or unattractive?" In this case, you have the choice to give greater value to the other person's opinion than your own, or you may simply recognize that he is expressing an opinion based on his belief system.

You could ask, "What makes you think that?" What if this person came from a tribe where the measure of a woman's beauty was the number of symbolic markings on her face? Then your "plain" face would not be perceived as attractive. So whether it is an insult or a compliment, this is only a reflection of what the other person thinks. Even if the words are said by someone who intentionally says hurtful things, it's not about you.

Jane's story shows how she avoided taking things personally. Jane was presenting at a conference and had put great effort into covering the salient points. After her presentation, several colleagues validated her hard work and spoke highly of the lecture. As she was packing up, a woman approached and told Jane that she thought the presentation was irrelevant and superficial. Jane breathed, paused, and then advised the lady that it would require considerable time for her to respond appropriately. As the woman walked away, Jane smiled, recognizing that everyone has an opinion.

Jane recited these affirmations: "May I not be elated by praise. May I not be offended by insult." Jane understood that her colleagues' compliments were expressions of their kindness based on their perception of the lecture. In like manner, the woman's disapproval reflected her own negativity. Jane could appreciate the validation from her colleagues and observe the woman's criticism without any inflation or deflation of ego. She would not attach her feelings to the roller coaster of other people's opinions.

This is not to be taken to the other extreme, like people with the "wreck a compliment syndrome." These are the ones who automatically discount a compliment. For example, upon hearing "You look very nice. That's a perfect color for you," the immediate reaction would be "This old thing! I meant to throw it out years ago." A simple "Thank you" keeps the focus on the other person's kindness.

In the movie *Roadhouse*, the character Dalton, played by Patrick Swayze, is trying to convince the bouncers of the bar about the importance of not taking anything personally. One of them asks, "What if someone calls your mother a whore? How can you not take that personally?" Dalton responds with humor, "Well, is she?" You may feel that someone is trying to put you down, but you do not have to let them take you down.

All the water is the world cannot drown
you unless it gets inside you.
—Eleanor Roosevelt

There is the story of a cab driver who had his fair share of being exposed to rude people. On one occasion, he swerved to avoid an accident, and the driver of the other car sprang out of his car and started shouting at the cab driver. The cab driver smiled and waved, and the irate driver went back to his car, shouting that the cab driver was making him late for work. The passenger in the cab expressed his amazement at the cab driver's composure, in staying calm and friendly. The cab driver explained it this way: "First of all, you have to learn to not take it personally. Many people are like garbage trucks; they run around with garbage, and when they are filled up with resentment, disappointment, anger, and fear, they try to dump it on others. You learn not to let them dump their garbage on you, and you make sure you don't spread the garbage around to others in your life. You pray for them and wish them well." The cab driver would not allow some stranger to ruin his day.

Take everything personally, and you are guaranteed to be miserable.

This story shows that people may have their perception of you, but that is not you. I had a college assignment and replicated a research study. No one, neither the presenter nor the students, was informed that they were participating in a study. The results would show whether people will be influenced by what they are told about someone, even before actually meeting the person.

I invited a physician to make a presentation and advised the class that we were having a guest speaker. Students were instructed to read the introduction of the presenter quietly and not discuss this.

When he arrived, no formal introduction was made. All the students were asked to pay attention, and they would be required to complete a survey at the end of the presentation. Two questionnaires with identical questions were randomly distributed. Half of the students received the form that introduced the presenter as a well-respected chiropractor with a successful practice, who was popular with his staff and patients because of his caring nature. Remaining students got the other form that described him as a famous chiropractor who had excellent skills, but his staff found him rude and arrogant, and many patients complained about his abrupt manner.

The intention was to determine if the same professional making the presentation, with the only difference being what the participants read about him on the form, would bring similar evaluations of the information given and the presenter himself.

The scores showed that a significant number of the students rated the presenter higher or lower depending on which form they had been given. The conclusion was that the positive introduction made a measurable difference. At the debriefing, students were dismayed that their unconscious judgment of the presenter had been influenced by the negative personality traits they had read at the beginning. This serves as a good reminder that you do not have to be a slave to other people's opinions. It's not about you anyway.

Sometimes, this message comes closer to home. There is often a person in the family who impulsively says hurtful things and later expects everyone to "just get over it."

Betty shared about what she learned from a distressing conversation with her cousin, Polly. Betty had witnessed the demeaning words that Polly inflicted on other family members, yet she felt that Polly would never say anything like that to *her*. One day, during a telephone conversation, it was Betty's turn to receive a spiteful attack. She was caught completely off guard, and the pain was so intense she ended the conversation and sat in stunned silence.

Betty decided to call Polly back to let her know how

painful her words had been. Polly was still armed after the interruption and ready to keep firing. Betty quickly terminated the call. Betty felt the flow of hot tears as she experienced the aftershock of this hateful encounter. Bewildered, she kept asking herself, "Why would Polly be so hateful to *me*?"

Then one day, Betty learned, through her own therapy and reading, that she had a choice all along. She could not control what Polly said, but she could process what she heard. Polly callously said hurtful things to everyone, and Betty did not have to personalize the unkindness.

With this change of perception, Betty came away with some lessons. Her first lesson was the reminder that hurtful words belonged to the speaker. Another lesson was that her first thought was automatic, but Betty could control what she did with the thought. She could ruminate over the words and feel offended, or she could stop, breathe, explore, and release. She could reflect on the words and determine what, if anything, to keep and what to reject.

Just as Betty would not allow anyone to dump trash in her living room, she would no longer allow anyone to dump verbal trash in her brain. However, if she happened to lose her favorite ring while cleaning up the kitchen, she would not hesitate to search through the garbage. Once she found her ring, she would retrieve it, wash it off, and then throw out the trash. In like manner, Betty could look for and validate any helpful advice—for example, "Thank you for suggesting that I wear the gray suit to the interview"—and dismiss any accompanying insults, such as "You're so clueless you would probably wear something totally unsuitable." Betty felt a new sense of freedom from the negativity of others.

It is most important not to confuse this with stuffing feelings and pretending they do not hurt, only to have them build up and explode later. This is about recognizing that you are defined by your own words, not by the other person's words. When you realize that the hurtful sarcasm coming from the other person is an expression of pain and anger, you can choose not to take it personally and thus not be injured by it.

Every moment that you spend upset, in despair,
in anguish, angry, or hurt because of the behavior
of anybody else in your life, is a moment in
which you've given up control of your life.
—Wayne Dyer

A great example of not taking anything personally is the story of the Buddha, who endured three days with a fellow traveler who constantly insulted the Buddha by calling him a fool and other disparaging words. Toward the end of the three days, the traveler could not understand how it was that the Buddha responded in a loving manner no matter what unkind thing the traveler said. When questioned, the Buddha replied, "If someone offers you a gift, and you do not accept that gift, to whom does the gift belong?" Then, the traveler understood.

If someone's "gift" to you is an insult, and you do not accept it, to whom does the insult belong? The insult remains with the person who tried to hurt you. You have no need to be hurt or angry since the insult does not belong to you; it belongs to the person who offered it to you. You realize that the hurtful words are reflections of the other person's internal pain monster, which you can witness without absorbing any of it.

Similarly, a gift of a compliment can be viewed as words from a kind person who wants to be validating. You can appreciate the person's praise without letting this flatter you. Others' opinions are still not about you, and you don't have to be a yo-yo by feeling flattered one day or offended the next by everyone who shows up in your life. These are the choices you make, consciously or unconsciously. As Margaret Thatcher said, "If my critics saw me walking over the Thames, they would say it was because I couldn't swim."

You may have heard the age-old jingle "sticks and stones can break your bones, but names will never harm you." This is possible when you don't take things personally. You can simply let hurtful remarks pass right through you. Think of a time when someone waved and you spontaneously waved back even though you didn't recognize the person. Then you discovered that he was not waving at you but at someone behind you.

Consider a cloud; if someone were to shoot at the cloud, the bullet would simply pass through, and the cloud would be unharmed. You can choose to do the same with a verbal attack: just let it pass through, offering no resistance as it goes away.

It's been said that if you were bitten by a snake, it is the lingering poison, not the bite, that causes the greater harm. Awareness can deflect the toxic words and keep you aligned with your commitment to give and receive only good things. Jesus's advice to "turn the other cheek" could be interpreted as "turn the other cheek and let it flow past you."

> Care about what other people think and
> you will always be their prisoner.
> —Lao Tzu

There is an old story about the people in a small, remote village and their highly respected healer who lived on the outskirts of town. He lived a quiet, reclusive life. The villagers often came to him for guidance, and he shared with them his wisdom.

A beautiful young girl in the village became pregnant.

She kept this secret to herself as long as she could and then realized that she could wait no longer to tell her parents. She was filled with fear at their reaction and the reaction of the other people in the village. She determined that the only way to escape from the harsh consequences was to tell them that the father of her child was, in fact, the healer.

Upon receiving the news, the girl's parents became outraged, and this was echoed by the other villagers as word spread swiftly throughout the village. The whole town stormed out to the healer's cottage and proceeded to unleash their accusations on him. When they had said every cruel thing that they could think of, they finally demanded that he have to take responsibility for the child and that when the child was born, the child would be brought to him. The healer listened in silence, and when they finally ran out of words, they waited expectantly for his response. He simply said, "Ah-so."

Months later, the child was born and taken to the healer. A year went by, and the young girl was overwhelmed with her guilt. She deeply regretted the turmoil she had caused with her lie, for indeed the father of her child was a young man in the village. So, she went to her parents and confessed her wrongdoing. Mortified, the entire village went back to the healer's cabin at the edge of town, apologized at length, and asked him to return the child to his mother. They waited anxiously for his response. The healer presented them with the child, who appeared healthy and happy. The young girl received the child gratefully into her arms. The healer looked at them and said, "Ah-so."

When the time comes that you feel that your integrity has been unjustly attacked, you will be able to maintain your peace and dignity by knowing that anyone can ruin your reputation, but no one can ruin your character.

Confidence is not "They'll like me." Confidence
is "I'll be okay if they don't."
—Christina Grimmie

This story shows that your perception can be the cause
of your pain, even when there was no intent to offend you.

> Then one said to Jesus, "Look, Your mother
> and Your brothers are standing outside,
> seeking to speak with You." But He answered
> and said to the one who told Him, "Who
> is My mother and who are My brothers?"
> And He stretched out His hand toward His
> disciples and said, "Here are My mother and
> My brothers! For whoever does the will of My
> Father in heaven is My brother and sister and
> mother." (Matthew 12:47–50 NKJV)

Mary had traveled many arduous miles to see her son,
Jesus, after a long separation. Based on her perception, she
could have felt dismissed and offended by Jesus's response
on hearing of their arrival. Mary knew her son well. When
minutes later Jesus greeted her with open arms, "Mother," she
was able to enjoy the embrace. Instead of taking it personally
and feeling slighted, she understood that Jesus was making
the point that they were all brothers and sisters, sons and
daughters. His response had nothing to do with the love of
his mother or his happiness to see her.

Oscar's story is another example. At the end of one of our
therapy sessions, Oscar's wife said that the most important
thing she had learned was that Oscar's behavior was never
intended to hurt her, and this problem was not her fault.
"Even though he told me many times that it was not about

me, everything was more painful when I believed he did not care, didn't love me, or blamed me."

Oscar's wife learned that when his intense craving was triggered, he did not think about her, his family, his job, his home, or even his own life; the only all-consuming compulsion was seeking the next drink or drug. Later that evening, Oscar asked to speak with me after the family group. He shared that the most valuable benefit of his treatment program was his gratitude that his wife now understood that his problem had never been about her, even when he had used the excuse of blaming her. He accepted that only when his addiction was addressed through a physical, emotional, and spiritual process would he be able to move forward to sobriety, regain his life, and repair their relationship. Whatever the outcome, Oscar's wife would no longer have to prolong her suffering by taking it personally.

> What others say and do is a projection of their
> own reality, their own dream. When you are
> immune to the opinions and actions of others,
> you won't be the victim of needless suffering.
> —Miguel Ruiz, *The Four Agreements*

Key Points

- Breathe.
- Listen as others share their opinions.
- Know that what they say about you is only their perception of you.
- View praise or insult as a gift, which you can accept or not. Either way, it is not about you.
- Anyone can ruin your reputation, but no one can ruin your character.

Choose to be inspired by the cab driver, Mary, the healer, and the Buddha. Don't take things personally. As the detached observer, you can calmly decide to accept only the things that nurture your soul. With practice, you can relinquish the exhausting behavior of people-pleasing and strive to be the best you.

CHAPTER 7

❦

Guard against Defensiveness

If we can drop our defensive posture and listen,
it gives us power—power to be influenced
and power to influence others.
—David Marcum and Steven Smith

It is probably safe to say that every one of us has been in a situation where we became defensive. This can happen for a host of reasons; the person's tone might have been aggressive or condescending, the timing could have been off, or perhaps we might not be in the right frame of mind to hear the message. When the question was asked, "What makes listening so hard?" many replied, "Being defensive!"

By raising your awareness of your emotional state—feeling overwhelmed, embarrassed, fearful, sad, or irritated—you can process these feelings first in order to clear the mind. When you witness and release distracting thoughts and feelings, you can become open to the guidance being offered.

Everyone and everything around you is your teacher.
—Ken S. Keyes Jr.

Here is a version of a popular Zen story. "Once, a university professor traveled halfway around the world to study with a Zen master, to open his mind to enlightenment.

While the master quietly served tea, the professor talked continuously about Zen, his thoughts, his ideas, and his speculations. As he rambled on and on, the master poured the professor's cup to the brim, until it began to overflow and run all over the floor. The professor watched what was happening until he could no longer restrain himself. He shouted, 'Stop, stop! The cup is full; you can't get any more in.' The master stopped pouring and said, 'You are like this cup; you are full of ideas about Zen. You come and ask for teaching, but your cup is full; I can't put anything in. Before I can teach you, you'll have to empty your cup.'"

When we are impressed with our own ideas, opinions, and self-importance, we may feel insecure when approached with new ideas. Thus we become defensive rather than attempting to see things from a different perspective. When defensiveness arises, important communication is lost.

Our bodies provide us with a detectable internal alarm system. When we are in tune with our bodies, we can recognize what is about to happen. The attendees at several lectures were asked, "Where in your body do you experience feeling defensive?" Some responses were, "In my chest, it feels tight," "In my stomach," "I find myself clenching my teeth," "My shoulders tense up." Stop for a moment and reflect on where you feel it in your body when you are becoming defensive.

A helpful acronym adapted from Al-Anon is JADE: justify, argue, defend, excuse. If you find yourself doing any of these, you may be feeling threatened or resisting new information. Chances are you will be participating in a conversation where everyone is talking and no one is listening—undoubtedly a waste of time and energy!

This story shows the importance or recognizing and removing defensiveness. Jerry and Mary had been working on improving their communication. On the way home from a social event, Mary shared with Jerry her observation of a comment he had made during the evening. She felt it may have been unintentionally upsetting to the other person. Jerry's immediate reaction was to defend his behavior. He expressed his extreme discomfort that anyone would be disturbed by anything he said. Perhaps in future he should not speak at all! Mary waited as Jerry vented his thoughts and feelings.

> Me thinks thou dost protest too much.
> —William Shakespeare (adapted)

When he became quiet, she reminded him that this was only her perception of the event, and her intention was to have him consider how this could have felt for the other person. Jerry listened and then processed what Mary had said, and he was eventually able to see the situation from another perspective. He was surprised how quickly he had become defensive with someone as loving and caring as Mary. He thanked Mary for her calm and gentle way of guiding him.

An activity that can provide opportunities for you to guard against defensiveness is ballroom dancing for partners. Often it is much easier to take constructive criticism from the instructor, simply because he teaches you to become a better dancer. When the instructor has the people skills to do this effectively, this makes the lessons more beneficial. The real challenge is how partners can take suggestions from each other. Once you let go of defensiveness, you can discuss the suggestions openly without any need to control, and the common goal is to improve individually and as partners.

In this story, Gene and Marlene chose cooperation over defensiveness. Marlene was a more advanced dancer, and Gene said that this was helpful for him, especially when they practiced between lessons. United by the goal of improving, they were able to give and receive helpful directions. For example, Marlene was continuously working on improving her posture, an important aspect of ballroom dancing, and Gene was often unaware when he would frown or pout during a more difficult step that he had not yet mastered. They agreed to point out to each other whenever they fell back into old behaviors. Their instructor often validated them for their attitude, as there were many other couples who were very critical of each other, and dancing became a struggle or competition rather than fun.

We all begin our education by being amateurs,
and in the real sense of the word we must remain amateurs.
—Holst, 1921

The root of the word "amateur" comes from the French word for love, and it is important to maintain the love of whatever you are doing and not have it be overshadowed by elitism or ego. Whatever you are aspiring to accomplish, recognizing and deactivating your defensiveness allows you to listen to the feedback, determine what is helpful, and apply the new learning accordingly.

For the ego (false self), defensiveness is an automatic reaction. The description of the ego given by Sogyal Rinpoche in *The Tibetan Book of Living and Dying* is captured in the essence of this paragraph: "Two people have been living in you all of your life. One is the ego, garrulous, demanding, hysterical, calculating; the other is the hidden spiritual being, whose still voice of wisdom you have only rarely heard or attended to."

Ego keeps you separate and unconnected. Whether you feel superior or inferior, entitled or undeserving, you do not want anyone to see behind your mask of fear. Ego can be easier to recognize in the person who boasts of being smarter or better, yet it exists in the one who presents as the most self-effacing person. In either case, feelings of being different, threatened, or judged are being fueled by fear.

Lack of self-confidence makes it uncomfortable to listen to suggestions without feeling that your ideas are being discounted. When you catch yourself shutting out information, you can identify the inner turmoil and resistance. You can become stronger emotionally and open the path to new information. Awareness is key, and the level of self-confidence will affect the receptivity/defensiveness. Gender can play a role: man speaking to man, woman to man, man to woman, woman to woman. The differences may dissolve in correlation with enlightenment. The more you learn, the more open-minded you become.

> Fear is the mortar that holds together
> the wall of defensiveness.
> —David Marcum and Steven Smith

There are highly regarded, learned teachers/scholars whose method of teaching is using questions on the part of the students, from which discussion can arise. They explore the probing, insightful questions that reveal their students' depth of understanding. Free of the constraints of ego, the teachers listen openly rather than being defensive or dismissive of their students.

Einstein, for example, did not respond well to the authoritarian style of a teacher whose prognosis for Einstein was, "He will never get anywhere."

In contrast, Einstein was greatly influenced by his Greek teacher, the brilliant mathematician, Konstantinos Karatheodoris, whom Einstein held in the highest regard. Karatheodoris's cooperation and communication with Einstein for the theory of relativity is imprinted in the letters they exchanged, which now are exhibited in the museum Karatheodoris in Komotini.

With their wealth of knowledge, confident teachers encourage dialogue, cognizant that the role of teacher/student can switch back and forth in the journey of discovery. There is no place for defensiveness or ego in this type of interchange.

Change is the end result of all true learning.
—Leo Buscaglia

Key Points

- Breathe.
- Quiet the mind and listen.
- Recognize any telltale signs of resistance in your body.
- Be patient as you strive to understand.
- Be open-minded.
- Share your perspective if the other person is receptive.
- Accept and incorporate what is helpful.
- People who ask questions are always learning and growing.

When you know that you are enough and you have enough, you discover that defensiveness can impede growth. Become aware of how easily you can let fear block the love and prosperity you deserve. Focus on the strengths in yourself and others and identify, accept, and work on changing any negative traits. Explore information with an open mind and guard against defensiveness.

CHAPTER 8

Relinquish the Need to Be Right

Would you rather be right, or would you rather be happy?
—From *A Course in Miracles*

The need to be right reveals the yearning for external validation. The compulsive need to be right can be insatiable, and the intense surge of adrenalin is fleeting. At the end of a heated dispute, one may be declared the winner. In terms of their relationship, both will lose if this creates disconnection.

It can be challenging when someone requests your feedback and immediately contradicts your response. In this type of situation, you need to ask yourself, "Is this person seeking information, or is this an invitation to debate?" This will determine whether you decide to invest any more energy in the conversation.

> To argue with a man who has renounced the use
> and authority of reason, and whose philosophy
> consists in holding humanity in contempt, is
> like administering medicine to the dead, or
> endeavoring to convert an atheist by scripture.
> —Thomas Paine, *The American Crisis*

There are times when the situation is quite trivial. Sally was looking forward to getting together with her good friend Bobby.

He had called to let her know that he was in a new relationship, and he wanted to introduce her. They met at the South Miami Arts Festival. As they strolled along, it soon became evident that Bobby's girlfriend was an authority on almost everything. They approached a booth where the photographer's work displayed exotic locations. Bobby's girlfriend pointed out a photograph that she recognized as an area on a Hawaiian island. Sally mentioned that it looked like a famous area in St. Lucia. Bobby's girlfriend fired back immediately. "No! This was absolutely taken in Hawaii. My family vacationed in the islands." Sally decided that it really wasn't important, and she would simply let it go. Bobby's girlfriend kept on. "I'll prove I'm right. I'll ask the photographer."

When questioned, the photographer assured Bobby's girlfriend that the photograph was taken of the majestic St. Lucia Pitons. She persisted, "Well, I'm pretty sure this looks like the mountains in Hawaii, and I've been there!"

The photographer spoke slowly. "This is said to be the most photographed site in the Caribbean, St. Lucia's iconic mountain pair. I took this photograph, and I have never been to Hawaii." He saw her frown and added, as if in consolation, "People often compare St. Lucia's lush foliage with Hawaii."

Bobby's girlfriend shrugged and left the booth. Sally thought of the joke about the young man who searched the world and finally found Miss Right, and later, to his dismay, discovered that her first name was Always! Sally hoped that Bobby was paying attention.

> Those who think they know it all have
> no way of finding out they don't.
> —Leo Buscaglia

This story shows how insufficient information can activate defensiveness. Consider the situation where Beth and

Mary agree to meet at the Macy's store in Dadeland Mall in Miami. They establish the time to meet, and both arrive right on time and anxiously begin consulting their watches. A phone call reveals that they are in fact both on time, they are both at Macy's, but Beth is at the home store at one end of the mall, and Mary is at the location in the middle of the mall. The next few minutes could be spent arguing about who was wrong and justifying the reason that each person chose the right location. Beth says, "I was at the Lancôme counter, where we always meet when we come to the mall."

Mary replies, "I was at the home store, because we were going to look at the luggage I need for my trip." Depending on the intensity of the need to be right, they can have this ruin their time together or laugh it off and agree to be more specific in the future.

Another great example can be witnessed any day of the week at the airport. Two people may have been apart and look forward to being together again. The drive to the airport increases the anticipation. As often happens, there could be a delay, and the magic evaporates as an argument ensues for reasons such as "You came to the wrong terminal, and you made me wait for an hour," or "I always pick you up on the departures level. How was I supposed to know you were waiting on the arrivals level?" This heated argument could continue all the way home and derail the loving reunion. In either scenario, when the focus shifts from attributing blame to looking for ways to improve communication, the relationship can be strengthened.

Accepting responsibility will empower you to consider what can be done differently next time so there will be less room for error. When, despite your best efforts, miscommunication happens, you can simply learn from the experience. In this way, you relinquish the need to be right and cultivate the desire to communicate. In any communication, you are creating either distance or intimacy. When you focus on convincing the other person to agree with your opinions, you are creating distance. When you focus on understanding where the other person is coming from, you are creating intimacy.

There was a similar misunderstanding when Bill arrived at the airport around midnight after a long flight. He called his son, Ian, and told him "I have arrived." When an hour went by and his son was not there to pick him up, he called him again to inquire what was happening. His son replied, "Oh, I thought you said, 'I have a ride.'" In this case, they were able to laugh about it and take into consideration that they were both tired and next time would confirm that what was said had actually been understood.

> Love is a game two can play and both win.
> —Eva Gabor

People will die to be right. People will kill to be right. History reveals the devastating consequences when this need to be right manifests in areas such as politics, religion, race, and sexual orientation. News of atrocities is beamed right through the television screen into our homes, from distant lands and from our own backyard. There are reports of children being brainwashed to hate and to commit heinous crimes against the "evil" enemy, with promises of great rewards in the afterlife. These misguided young people go on to justify the vicious acts they later carry out. There are other shocking instances of distorted thinking, like the irate man who believed that abortion was wrong and felt it was right to take the life of a doctor outside an abortion clinic, the father who felt duty bound to kill his daughter to save the family disgrace when his daughter refused to marry the man to whom she had been promised at birth, or the road rage from traffic infractions that becomes deadly.

When you are driven by the need to be right, your opinions restrict you. The intense desire to defend your position leaves no room for growth. The need to be right can make you try to show how much smarter you are than everyone else. Belittling someone is a way to prove that you deserve recognition. Your recurring thoughts, from a monologue, dialogue, or entire committee, keep you guarded and fearful.

German physician Werner Forssmann faced this type of opposition. When he was still an intern, he theorized the basics of cardiac catheterization. The catheter, he surmised, could be used to ferry drugs needed for cardiac resuscitation directly into the heart. His superiors adamantly dismissed the idea. "Unbelievable, impossible!" His boss forbade him to continue.

It took all the courage and determination of this young surgical resident to use exactly that means in order to achieve one of clinical cardiology's greatest advances. Werner Forssmann conducted the experiment on himself in 1929. He anesthetized his own lower arm and opened the antecubital vein in his elbow, inserted a small metal tube into his bloodstream, and watched on a fluoroscope screen as it progressed up his arm and toward his heart. He then walked down the hall and up two flights of stairs to have an x-ray taken, showing the catheter in his right auricle, near the atrium of his heart. Learning of the significance of his discovery, the popular press acclaimed his work.

The drive to discredit Forssmann's accomplishment was so strong that the medical establishment condemned him as crazy, scorning him and ignoring his work for over a decade. The experiment paved the way for many types of heart studies. Much to his amazement, Forssmann was later awarded with the Nobel Prize in 1956.

One of the truest signs of maturity is the ability to
disagree with someone while still remaining respectful.
—DaveWillis.org

Your willingness to be wrong and imperfect involves
accepting how much you do not know, an expression of your
strength and self-esteem. You recognize how your beliefs
affect your life and others. You are open to all teachers, ready
to incorporate new information. Each experience prompts the
question, "What did I learn?"

Confidence comes not from always being
right, but from not fearing to be wrong.
—Peter McIntyre

In healthy relationships, each can explore an experience
openly and strive to walk away with a deeper understanding
of the other, or simply agree to disagree without being
disagreeable. As often happens, when the discord is revisited
later, they realize that they were not discussing the same
issue. They were unable at the time to listen with caring
curiosity. Each was too intensely focused on being heard,
rather than striving to understand the other. Precious time
is wasted trying to unravel the misunderstandings that were
caused by the need to be right.

Imagine being in a room that has two windows; one
faces the vast ocean, complete with white sand beaches
and picturesque palm trees, and the other window faces
beautiful mountains with lush vegetation. As you gaze out
your window, you share what you are witnessing, while
the other person looks out the other window and insists
that you are wrong, because the view is quite different.
You waste the present moment trying to convince each
other that the view from your window is the right one. You

do not listen to each other, because you have to be right, and that means the other person has to be wrong. As the comedian said, "Don't confuse me with the facts. I already made up my mind." When you remain stuck with the view from your window, you miss the opportunity to expand your horizon.

Perhaps for future conversations, you might calmly look out the other person's window and invite this person to look out your window. This flexibility can increase rapport, as you look for similarities rather than differences, understanding and cooperation rather than arrogance and competition.

Every person that you meet knows something you don't.

—Bill Nye

Open-minded people are able to participate in brainstorming, giving and receiving innovative ideas, and everyone benefits. When questioned about a belief, they are willing to explore their thinking and discover another perspective.

After listening to the earlier story about Forssmann, a physician shared with the writer that he thought that Forssmann was a urologist, not a cardiologist. They discovered that Forssmann was discouraged by the fierce opposition and switched to urology. They were both right, without either of them having the need to be right, and they learned something new.

If you state that the world is round and a close-minded person remains adamant that the world is flat, whether you argue or let go of the need to be right does not change the fact. So why waste precious energy in a senseless debate? There is an important difference between wanting to be clear and needing to be right. You want to be heard and understood;

you do not need to have the other person openly concede that you are right.

When you decide that you want to be free of the need to be right, you get many opportunities to practice this new concept. You take a breath, observe if you are feeling triggered to engage, and determine whether there is any value in pursuing the topic. If you see that the other person only wants to be right, you can go to curiosity and perhaps learn something. The other person may act out their frustration when you do not continue the dispute. Be vigilant. If it gets to the point that the conversation is taking your peace to no avail, find a tactful way to end it. Each similar interchange will reinforce your sense of empowerment.

Those who danced were thought to be quite insane
by those who could not hear the music.
—Unknown

Key Points

- Breathe.
- Determine if this is a conversation or a debate.
- Ask yourself, "How important is it?"
- Remember, facts remain unchanged, no matter who is right or wrong.
- Understand that you can both be right.
- Be curious about what the other person is saying.
- Clarify if you are both discussing the same issue.
- Welcome an opportunity to expand your knowledge.
- If the other person is driven by the need to be right, you can save energy and simply stop talking.
- "Would you rather be right, or would you rather be happy?"

When being right or wrong no longer enhances or diminishes your self-esteem and self-worth, you are free to communicate your thoughts and feelings in a clear, dispassionate manner. There is no need to force or convince the other person to agree with your beliefs. You are happy to share what you know, and then you just stop talking. You clear the way to being open and receptive to other ideas and concepts. You are intrigued by all the things you have yet to learn.

CHAPTER 9

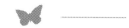

Be Direct. Be Kind.

Be kind whenever possible. It is always possible.
—Dalai Lama

Relationships often begin with hopes and dreams for a fulfilling life together. Over time, many forget that a relationship is like a beautiful garden that needs to be cared for. You may become complacent and allow other priorities to become more important: work, finances, parental and household tasks, comparison with other people's successes, and so on. One day, you look out the window and wonder what happened to your lovely garden, overrun with the weeds of neglect.

Communication can be the most affected area. You speak to each other with little regard, believing that loving each other means you will tolerate thoughtless remarks or indifference. You think your loved ones should know what you mean, even at times when you speak carelessly before engaging your brain.

This can manifest in different ways. Too often, a person who grew up in a critical, toxic family learned to say mean and spiteful things, followed by laughter to disguise the needless pain and hurt. He would then carry this pattern into the next generation and become a poor role model for his own children. When the hurt was too harsh to be concealed,

71

damage control would be, "You know I didn't really mean that. I was just angry," or "I had a bad day," or "I was just joking," or "You're mean to me sometimes too." These excuses will not repair the damage because these feelings have been stored in that automatic recorder in the brain. These words can't be deleted. What do you want your loved ones to remember?

Bob and Helen had one of their awful fights late one night. Their children retreated to their rooms and tried to drown out the ugliness with music or TV. They could never understand how their parents could be so mean to each other. The next morning, Helen noticed that their recording device had been left on. She was curious. As she listened, she recognized that this was a recording of their vicious fight. She was appalled at the fierce, hurtful words. She backed it up again and, one by one, erased all her replies. The next time the recording was played, only Bob's portion of the argument remained.

What if someone did that with your arguments? There would be no way to justify your reactions by saying, "It was his fault; he was mean to me first." You would have to take full responsibility for what you said. A person may feel they are controlling the situation by being louder and meaner, whereas the opposite is true. The only real control is self-control, strengthened by a commitment to be able to stand behind your spoken words. The moment the discussion moves from logic to emotion, it is time to pause. Silence reminds you that your words are a reflection of you, and you feel empowered by your restraint.

There is a great analogy that when you squeeze an orange, you will always get orange juice. When you get squeezed in a stressful situation, whatever you say reveals the pain or joy you have inside. You can listen and reflect on everything you say as you continue the work on your personal growth. You have no control over what others say. Their hurtful attacks are expressions of the pain and fear they carry inside their hearts. Biting criticism can only come from someone who is filled with negativity and low self-worth.

> For the mouth speaks what the heart is full of.
> —Luke 6:5 (NIV)

The aggressor will often say that he gets irritated and says spiteful things, but then he is over it five minutes later. He never considers the residual effect of his wrath on the recipient. Later, when he attempts to have a conversation with a stoic, silent partner, the aggressor has no concept of the other person's smoldering pain. If you start off your day with a mean, negative conversation, it is unlikely that your partner will feel loved and appreciated at the end of the day. If you want to have an affectionate partner, this will require kind, loving communication. Change is possible when each is willing to discuss the dynamic in a calm manner and make a commitment to resolve underlying issues.

> Say what you mean, mean what you
> say and don't say it mean.
> —Al-Anon

Be direct and say what you mean. Identify your motive or intention. What message are you transmitting? Will this express your hope for a better relationship or are you simply venting your anger or frustration? If the latter is the case, you can find appropriate ways to express and release these feelings without causing more pain. Processing your anger with a therapist or trusted friend, or journaling can be effective ways to explore and release pent-up emotions. This will clear the path to honest communication.

The next stage requires the introspection to clarify that you really mean what you say. If you say, "I want to end this," does this reflect your true feelings or is this impulsive and meaningless? Is this a setup? Do you expect the other person to read between the lines and know that you really want your partner to say, "I want us to be together forever"? Can you stand behind your words with a resounding, "Yes, I really meant exactly what I said"?

Conscious effort to control the tone and choice of words will ensure that you don't say it meanly. It is interesting how later, when you repeat a conversation, the tone can be entirely different. "Gee, dear, all I said was, 'Can we do this another time? I'm tired.'" She responds, "That's definitely not the way you said it!" A comedian gave an amusing illustration of what you say and how you say it. You look at your date and say, "When I look into your eyes, time stands still," and you don't say, "You have a face that would stop a clock."

There was a similar exchange between Johnny and Cynthia at a therapy session. Handling finances was an ongoing issue. Cynthia had purchased a mop online for twenty-five dollars, and when asked how much it cost, she said, "Two hundred dollars," in an attempt to be amusing.

Johnny blurted out, "No way. Cynthia is too cheap to spend $200 on a mop." This hit a nerve since many of their arguments arose from Johnny's careless overspending. Johnny was invited to be validating by saying, "Cynthia is too frugal to waste $200 on a mop." He replied, "Yes, that's what I meant." Cynthia commented that she hoped he would consider this in future conversations.

If you value your time together and want a lasting relationship, you have to work on communication that is nurturing—expressing wishes or resolving issues peacefully. You will know you are on the wrong track when you have to go back and say, "I was just kidding." Life is too short to be wasted on hurting each other.

This story is about recognizing and changing a hurtful behavior. Rob and Alice decided to seek professional help when they recognized that their relationship was falling apart. One of the key issues that arose was Rob's constant sarcasm. He was, at first, surprised that Alice had such strong feelings about this issue. He thought that his sarcasm was humorous and harmless, and he believed that Alice had found this amusing. Alice, on the other hand, thought that Rob used sarcasm to distract from any serious conversations, and this would emerge at inappropriate times. She thought he was unaware of the facial expressions of those around him. She also felt as if people would look at her and wonder why she tolerated his insensitivity. Rob asked Alice to give him some examples. She had so many examples that he asked her to stop; he was beginning to understand what she had been trying to tell him for many years.

Rob agreed to work on changing this lifelong pattern. He asked Alice to gently point out whenever she saw him falling back into this old behavior. In the beginning, Rob was taken aback at how often Alice brought this to his attention. Over time, Rob worked through the feelings that triggered the sarcasm and found positive ways to express his thoughts. Their communication improved in direct relation to his commitment to be more open and honest. He also noticed that friends became more relaxed during their conversations, and humor became lighthearted and engaging.

Take the time to hear yourself before you speak and determine if your message sounds constructive or destructive. Speak as you would like to be spoken to and filter out anything you might regret later.

This story is about changing an old, negative pattern. Mary Beth shared about her parents who were planning to celebrate their fiftieth wedding anniversary. She was reluctant to return home and discussed this with her siblings. They shared about their discomfort when visiting their parents and realized that moving away had given them time and space for reflection. They had become more sensitive to their parents' chronic pattern of constantly making spiteful comments to each other under the guise of humor. When they gathered the courage to discuss this with their parents, they were braced for their parents' reaction.

Their parents' denial was eventually worn down, and they listened to Mary Beth and her siblings. This gentle, heartfelt guidance revealed to them how they inflicted their buried hurts and disappointments on each other. They agreed to find a healthy approach to resolving their issues. Their communication changed dramatically, and their fiftieth anniversary marked the beginning of a new chapter in their lives.

If speaking kindly to plants helps them grow,
imagine what speaking kindly to humans can do.
—Unknown

Being direct also means keeping your requests clear and simple. Consider a common occurrence at many family gatherings. After spending hours to prepare for the family holiday celebration dinner, Rosa is about to sit down when she realizes that the vegetable casserole was left in the oven. She sighs and complains, "Couldn't anyone have thought of bringing the casserole to the table?" with the unspoken thoughts, *After all that I have been doing all day, do I have to think of everything?* What is she asking? And who is "anyone"? She could keep it simple: "Mary, could you please bring the casserole from the oven?" When you are straightforward, you can eliminate the drama and make it easier on everyone.

Another example is entering a room and inquiring, "Is it hot in here?" An answer could be, "Oh, it doesn't feel hot to me." A direct request would be, "Would it be all right if I lowered the air-conditioning?" This concept applies equally to complaints. "You never take out the garbage" is a complaint that requires no direct action, versus turning a complaint into a request, "Would you please take out the garbage?" This suggestion often brings the rebuttal, "Well, I shouldn't have to ask him to take out the garbage!" This presents a choice: would you rather complain about the shoulds and be miserable or simply make a request? Being direct in a kind way contributes to understanding and action and is reinforced with an expression of gratitude. "Thanks for taking out the garbage."

When a parent was encouraged to thank her teenage son for taking out the garbage, her reply was, "Well, that's what he's supposed to do. Why should I thank him for that?" For her, it was much easier to nag and scold her son when he didn't take care of his tasks. The next question to her was "And how's that working for you?"

When you are mindful of your feelings and your motive, you express your desires or concerns thoughtfully.

Key Points

- Take a breath.
- Clarify what you want to say. Say what you mean, mean what you say.
- Check tone and content. Don't say it meanly.
- Is this direct and kind? Is it kind, is it necessary, is it true?

- What are you hoping to accomplish? What is your goal?
- Is this courteous? Will you feel good about your conversation later?
- Will this conversation strengthen the relationship?

When you speak with the intention of being helpful, not hurtful, your message will be hopeful, not hateful. Are you courteous with acquaintances but thoughtless with your loved ones? Elevate the importance of courtesy in all your interactions by treating others as you would like to be treated. Courteous behavior is love in action. Approach issues in a direct way, keeping the focus on the goal of mutual support and connection. Standing at the stern of a ship, watching the wake, can be a reminder of the wake that is left behind from what you said. What if this was your last conversation with this person? Strive to be kind in word and deed.

CHAPTER 10

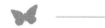

Be Aware of the Power of Your Words

> Knowing that words can create happiness or
> suffering, I am committed to speaking truthfully
> using words that inspire confidence, joy, and hope.
> —Thich Nhat Hanh

Every word you think and every word you speak has an impact on your well-being and the well-being of the people around you. Catch any disempowering words, such as can't, never, always, impossible, should. Whenever you think or speak these words, pay attention to the feelings these words elicit and the negative reinforcement that occurs. Fear can program your subconscious to ingest words that fuel anxiety.

> If you think you can or you think you can't, you're right.
> —Henry Ford

Consciously work toward becoming more vigilant about everything you incorporate in your thinking. Refuse to participate in a world in which people use words carelessly, hurting one another and damaging their relationships. Avoid gossip, which has been likened to a computer virus of the soul. Refrain from saying attacking words and also from accepting attacking words. Speak the language of possibility and focus on the best in yourself and others.

You may be surprised when someone tells you how he or she was influenced by something you said, and you realize the impact of a simple comment. This brings a deeper understanding of the need to be in control of every word you utter. If you look back and wish you could simply delete some distressing remark, you can use the experience to guide you to be more mindful in the present moment. A thoughtless word spoken when the other person was vulnerable can render needless pain and have far-reaching consequences. On the other hand, a compassionate word said in a similar situation can be healing and encouraging. In every conversation, you have the choice to plant seeds that can be helpful or hurtful. As Uncle Ben said in *Spiderman*, "With great power comes great responsibility." Always remember the power of your words.

The following is an interesting little story about the power of words. One day Thomas Edison came home and gave a paper to his mother. He told her, "My teacher gave this paper to me and told me to only give it to my mother."

His mother's eyes were tearful as she read the letter out loud to her child: "'Your son is a genius. This school is too small for him and doesn't have enough good teachers for training him. Please teach him yourself.'"

Many years after Edison's mother had died and he had become one of the greatest inventors of the century, one day he was looking through old family things. He came across a folded paper in the corner of a drawer in a desk. On the paper was written, "Your son is addled [mentally deficient]. We won't let him come to school anymore." Edison later wrote: "My mother was the making of me. She was always so proud of me, and I felt I had someone to live for, someone I must not disappoint."

Although there is no evidence that there was ever such a letter, Edison's mother's homeschooling had a big impact on him. Edison was dyslexic, and his teacher's rigid teaching method of having students memorize and recite lessons, and whipped for making mistakes, made school life a misery for Edison. This heartwarming story is worth retelling to highlight the power of a word and the responsibility to use words to empower self and others. Reassuring words can change a life.

This next story shows the insidious effects of negative patterns of communication. Betsy would tell anyone that she was happily married to Alfred. He was a congenial, unassuming man who had loved Betsy deeply from the time they first met. One day, Betsy listened in disbelief as her close friend Amy took the risk of asking a difficult question. "You know you are my dearest friend. What makes you say such belittling things to Alfred and then later switch to expecting his affection?" Betsy was immediately defensive, but later she began to reflect on her marriage. She got in touch with how self-absorbed she had become and how little she valued Alfred beyond his financial contribution to their affluent lifestyle. She decided to discuss this with Alfred. At first, Alfred assured her that everything was fine. As Betsy pressed him further, he haltingly disclosed that he had been distancing himself because it was becoming more difficult to feel close to her after each episode of her harsh remarks. He wondered if she realized how often she compared him unfavorably to their wealthy, high-achieving friends. He had been contemplating what his life would be like without having to be guarded all the time.

Betsy froze. Alfred had always seemed unaffected by anything she said. Memories of her parents' relationship came flooding back. She remembered all the times when her father had been so demeaning to her mother, how angry she became with him for his cruelty and with her mother for tolerating it. Betsy shuddered as she recognized how many of her father's negative traits she had incorporated, which had manifested in her total disregard of Alfred's feelings. Betsy was disheartened by who she had become, and angry with Alfred for passively being the victim.

Betsy and Alfred talked for hours and got in touch with how their early relationship had been filled with youthful goals. This was their turning point. Going forward, Betsy could learn to use words to restore, not destroy, their relationship. Alfred would express his feelings honestly. They began the process of renewal with a compassionate marriage counselor. They learned that the magic ratio, according to science, is five to one. This means that for every negative interaction during a conflict, a nurturing and happy marriage has five (or more) positive interactions.

Self-talk may be even more powerful. Is your self-talk gentle and encouraging, or is it punitive and discouraging? Our early messages in childhood can set the stage for our evolution. Our parents are our first gods, and their voices are almost hypnotic. The child raised with engaged, self-confident, and loving parents will have their internal voices play back the early motivating messages. The reverse is also true. The child raised with insecure, disengaged, and degrading parents may incorporate these disempowering words into his or her internal dialogue (parental introject). Later, these words may be projected onto other people to further reinforce feelings of worthlessness.

This brings to mind the poem "Children Learn What They Live" by Dorothy L. Nolte. This is an abridged 1959 version.

> If a child lives with criticism, he learns to condemn ...
> If a child lives with hostility, he learns to fight ...

If a child lives with fear, he learns to be apprehensive ...
If a child lives with pity, he learns to feel sorry for himself ...
BUT
If a child lives with tolerance, he learns to be patient ...
If a child lives with encouragement, he learns to be confident ...
If a child lives with acceptance, he learns to love ...
If a child lives with honesty, he learns what truth is ...
With what is your child living?

Sometimes our most harsh reactions are to our own actions, because of our intense need to be perfect. A handy word that can be used to delay and avoid a thoughtless reaction is "oops" (other opportunity to practice serenity), followed by a deep breath. Think about the times you made a simple mistake, like misplacing your keys or leaving home without something you needed or even breaking a glass, and your first reaction was to use words like "idiot" or "stupid" to chastise yourself. Instead, you could simply say "oops" and commit to being more focused. You can stop berating yourself with negative self-talk by interjecting the word "oops." This breaks the automatic sequence and gives you time to take that deep breath and put the event in perspective.

This story shows the importance of being vigilant about your self-talk. Jessie had gone through a devastating divorce. A year later, she gathered enough courage to go on a blind date after several exchanges online. She agreed to meet him at a restaurant. She waited nervously until she saw him approaching the table, the identifying red hankie in his lapel. As they were sipping coffee at the end of a delicious meal, he shared that he didn't think they were a fit and that it was not going to work out.

She felt sharp tears sting her eyes as she walked away. She sat in her car for a while and listened to her friend's comments. "Well, what did you expect? You're a middle-aged woman. You don't exactly look like a model. What would ever make you think that a good-looking guy like that would be interested in you?" Hearing this, one might ask, "How could any friend be so brutal? The fact is, those words did not come from a friend. They came from the voice inside her head, her own negative self-talk.

As Jessie processed this event, she understood that she had to break old self-defeating patterns. She had to be gentle and loving with herself and others. This change would be reflected in the words she used to positively shape her life.

> Make sure your own worst enemy is not
> living between your own two ears.
> —Laird Hamilton

"How important is it?" is a good question to ask yourself before you invest a disproportionate amount of energy in any situation. Each time you engage in negative self-talk, you send a shot of negativity to your subconscious to reinforce every bad feeling you have stored away. The harsh, inner critic in your head needs to be evicted and replaced with a loving motivator.

You discover the incalculable power of the words "I am ..." The next words will reveal to you and everyone the life you are creating. Damaging words such as "I am ... so clumsy/dumb, fat, poor, forgetful" project your reality. Research further reveals that people with symptoms of depression use an excessive amount of words that express negative emotions, such as sad, unhappy, and lonely. The important immediate step is to replace the negative self-talk with positive self-talk to benefit from the power of your words. Realizing that words can encourage or discourage, choose your words carefully.

A really sneaky word is "tired." The more often you repeat that you are tired, the more tired you will feel. Instead of verbalizing day after day how tired you are, shift your focus to the cause of your tiredness and determine what you can do differently. It isn't that all busy people are constantly tired, and others with less to do feel rested. You may need more balance in your life. Many folks create simple strategies, such as making the time for a power nap as a transition from professional to personal tasks. Any negative pattern can be broken, and harmful words can be replaced with uplifting ones, such as "I am focused on healthy living. I am developing better self-care. I am embracing new learning every day."

This is exciting news since the only person you can change is you. With the realization that your thoughts can impede or enhance your growth and happiness, you can begin the process of converting to positive self-talk. You stop damaging yourself and others with your words and choose instead to foster motivation and courage. You observe and discard any words that disrupt your peace.

Each year, hundreds of people on my address list receive an invitation to make a forty-day journey, to retreat and replenish during the Lenten season from Ash Wednesday to Easter Sunday. This can be a special period of self-reflection, spiritual practice, your religious practice, or simply a personal time-out to slow things down for contemplation. An important component is a negativity fast—when you endeavor to refrain from saying, thinking, or doing anything negative. Negative thoughts will come uninvited. You simply witness the thought and gently let it slip away and replace it with a positive one (catch it, check it, and change it). Consider this your invitation to join our negativity fast every year.

It's like learning a new language. You look for opportunities to interject positive words in your conversations. You surround yourself with others who speak and understand this engaging language. You can incorporate many acronyms, like ones in this book, and freely share them with friends along a similar path.

> Kind words are like honey—Sweet to the
> soul and healthy for the body.
> —Proverbs 16:24

Key Points

- Breathe.
- Process your thoughts before you speak.
- Observe any negative words and determine how positive words could be more effective.
- Remember to apply "oops" (other opportunity to practice serenity).
- In relationships or self-talk, remember the magic ratio of 5:1 positive to negative.
- Welcome opportunities to use words that are reassuring and supportive.

Slow down to reflect on the words you think and say to yourself and others. Interrupt and derail the mind's negative train of thought. Benefit from the research that shows how repeating positive words like peace, joy, love, and compassion will activate certain genes that lower your emotional and physical stress. Live each day fully, open and receptive to safe, loving relationships.

CHAPTER 11

Raise Self-Awareness to Guide Reframing

We either make ourselves miserable,
or we make ourselves strong.
The amount of work is the same.
—Carlos Castenada

Reframing is another effective coping strategy. Chances are, growing up you heard little gems such as "there is a reason for everything" and "everything passes, the good and the bad." Your willingness to take these messages to heart made a difference in how you interpreted challenges—whether you hung on to the suffering longer or you adapted and learned from the experience. This applies to little annoyances and to major issues. Reframing helps you seek and find options, and you move forward with a lighter heart. Later, you reflect on the personal growth that came as a result of going through these challenges.

Edna had inherited a lovely seascape picture that hung on a wall in her office. She really liked the picture despite the old, unappealing frame. One day, a client remarked to her that the beauty of the picture was diminished by the dilapidated frame. This comment resonated for her, and she decided to head over to the frame shop that afternoon. She chose a very attractive frame with a look of driftwood that really enhanced the picture. It was interesting to overhear the positive comments, as if everyone entering her office was seeing the picture for the first time. This is the concept of reframing; you put an old situation into a new frame to make a positive shift.

Joshua and Barbara applied this concept in a real-life situation. Joshua's job required a long commute to work each day. He came up with a solution that worked for him; he would ride his bike and then take the train to avoid the heavy rush hour traffic. He used that time on the train for reading or mindfulness. He became accustomed to this time with his own thoughts, and he could relax while someone else did the driving.

A few months later, Joshua's wife, Barbara, got a job in the building next to his, and she now faced a similar challenge of getting to work with a hectic commute. They decided that they would ride together. Joshua was back in the traffic and reverted to feeling more irritated each day. Barbara felt increasingly guilty that he had made this sacrifice for her and he was losing his peace because of her. Much of the time the ride was spent in silence, broken at times by Joshua's exclamations of frustration. They came to dread the drive each morning.

Then they remembered one of the tools they had learned, the art of reframing. They came up with the idea to use this time to catch up on the many things they were always too busy to explore. Sometimes they would listen to a pod cast and discuss what had resonated for each of them. They also took this time to make phone calls to family members, like Joshua's mother, which Joshua was often saying he should do.

Barbara transformed her feelings of guilt to gratitude for Joshua's kindness and for this special pocket of time together. Joshua was delighted to see how the traffic became only slightly annoying, especially once he acknowledged that he was part of the traffic. As a result, they actually looked forward to this time together at the beginning and end of each workday. Nothing outside had to change. Through reframing, they transformed distressing times into precious moments of connection.

> If you change the way you look at things,
> the things you look at change.
> —Wayne Dyer

There is a story of two men who carried bricks up a hill. When asked what they were doing, one replied, "I'm carrying bricks up the hill." The other answered, "I'm building a cathedral." They were doing the same activity, but only the second man brought meaning to his work. In so doing, he approached each day with enthusiasm, knowing that his gift would touch the hearts and lives of thousands of people. You can use this process to enrich your path every day.

Reframing works wonderfully when applied to current experiences. Reframing is also a great tool to resolve past painful events. From Plato, we learned that beauty lies in the eyes of the beholder. Thus, the designation of beauty states more about the observer than the observed. Similarly, meaning lies in the view of the perceiver. What happened to us, or whatever we said or did in the past is recorded according to our perception. This will influence the way we feel and act when triggered by similar events in the present. These memories are reflective of influences, such as our age at the time of the event, our tribe (i.e., family) values, culture, and environment. We reframe past experiences by challenging our chronic perceptions to bring new meaning and insight.

Millie's story is a good example of looking at a life experience with fresh eyes. When she was about six years old, she was delighted to be Daddy's girl, and she had mixed emotions when she learned that she was going to have a baby sister. She wasn't sure that she wanted to give up the attention of being an only child, "the little princess." A few months after her baby sister arrived, the atmosphere in the home changed. Her mother seemed sad most of the time. Her mother and father were often displeased with each other. Millie did her best to cheer everyone up, but her colicky baby sister added to the stress. One day, Millie's father sat down with her and explained that her mommy had gone away, because she could not bear to be a wife or mother any longer.

Millie did not understand what any of this meant, but deep down she knew it had to be her fault. In her little mind, she believed that something must be wrong with her, and that Daddy would be angry with her for making Mommy leave. Her baby sister went to live with her aunt and uncle, who had no children of their own, and Millie was taken care of by her nanny. Her father worked longer and longer hours and came home tired and depressed. She would often fall asleep on the couch waiting for him, and he would spend the evening drinking in front of the television. This experience, which was buried deep in her heart, had a great influence on her self-esteem and her inability to trust. She felt alone, unlovable, and unattractive.

At age twenty-four, Millie revisited this painful period of her life. She learned that her mother, who was only twenty years old at the time, left because of her own inability to cope with the pressures of being a parent and wife, as a result of her own dysfunctional childhood. Millie came to see that none of her "story" was true. She had not been the cause of her mother's unhappiness. Her father had not blamed her for her mother's leaving, nor had he punished her by sending her baby sister away. Her parents had done the best they could at the time and experienced their own guilt for not giving Millie the love she deserved.

Over time, Millie healed her relationship with her parents. She learned to reframe the experience by seeing two imperfect people who were ill-equipped to be parents. She was grateful for the loving nanny who had tried so hard to compensate for Millie's abandonment. She validated her own courage for taking responsibility for her pain, her feelings, her acceptance, and growth. She recognized that the past was a place to learn from, not a place to live. She was free to view life through a new lens.

There are endless opportunities to apply this tool. At a meditation group held at a park by the beach, participants ranged from first timers to experienced meditators. Beginning meditators often think that quiet is an integral part of meditation. During a brief introduction to meditation, they were encouraged to allow any sounds, such as a passing boat with loud music or conversations of people walking by, to simply become part of the meditation without any need to judge or be disturbed. At the end, many shared how they had been able to integrate all the distractions, and in fact when someone began playing his guitar right next to the group, they felt that this gentle music enhanced the experience. Thus, through the process of reframing, the meditation was beneficial.

> You gotta look for the good in the
> bad, the happy in your sad,
> the gain in your pain and what makes
> you grateful not hateful.
> —Karen Salmansohn

Self-awareness is the precursor to changing the internal dialogue through reframing.

You discover how your feelings shift when you choose one perspective over the other. You envision the light at the end of the tunnel even in the darkest times. Believing that you are moving toward the light sustains you in each moment and guides you to the potential blessing.

After taking the time to identify and understand the barriers to your well-being, you can use reframing to shift your focus to the possibilities to stimulate action and growth. Your new pattern of reframing will also unearth the gems that may be hidden or disguised as challenges. You can be aggravated because your neighbor's dog barks at night, or you can be grateful that you have the gift of hearing, which is verified when you hear the dog barking. You can simply let your ears hear what they hear without judgment. That is self-awareness and reframing.

> When I have a toothache, I discover that not having
> a toothache is a wonderful thing. That is peace.
> —Thich Nhat Hanh

Consider the story from the Bible (Samuel 1:17) about David, the young boy who faced the giant Goliath, armed only with a slingshot. One can imagine that the soldiers were saying, "He is so big. How can you possibly defeat him?" while David was thinking, *He is so big; I cannot miss him.* Your ability to use reframing will impact your life experience in profound ways.

> Sometimes God will put a Goliath in your life,
> for you to find the David within you.
> —Toby Mckeehan

Key Points

- Breathe.
- Explore the situation that is causing your discomfort.

- Recognize how your thinking is driving your feelings.
- Consider other ways of seeing the issue. Feedback from others can be helpful.
- Discover any hidden blessings and be grateful for them.
- Change the situation or change your perception.
- Let go of unnecessary suffering.

Reframing brings a deeper level of understanding that not getting what you want can bring you as much happiness as getting what you want. You recognize that you never see the whole picture. When you look out the window, you see one view. If you were to go up to the roof and look all around, you would have a wider view, and if you went up in a helicopter, the view would expand accordingly. Your awareness of the cause of your distress and your ability to reframe your situation will bring you the acceptance and peace you desire.

CHAPTER 12

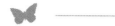

Shed the Burden of Judgment

Look beyond the story and see the Soul.
—Suggestion from Seane Corn

There is a popular saying, "Judging others does not define who they are; it defines who you are." Everyone has judged other people at some time, and usually without having all the facts. Whatever the reason for judging others—appearance, language, education, and endless other categories—judging is negative, opinionated, and separates you from others. Since no one knows more about every topic than any other person, no human being is superior, overall, to any other.

Judgment has a negative effect on your thoughts, emotions, and even your physical well-being. This can become a pervasive pattern, especially if you associate with other judgmental people. Judgment can get in the way of a peaceful and healthy lifestyle. Judging others fuels the fear of being judged by others.

Those who look for the bad in people will surely find it.
—Abraham Lincoln

Think about the effect of judgment as you read the following story ...

Rebecca tries to be a helpful person. She spends a great

deal of time at church, taking care of many of the behind-the-scenes activities, as well as regularly attending services. This particular Sunday morning, she arrived early, as usual, and sat in her favorite pew. She relaxed as she watched other parishioners arrive. Just as the service was about to begin, she saw a young girl rush in and sit at the end of the closest pew.

Rebecca looked at her and immediately frowned with great disdain. She disapproved of the way this young woman was dressed. Clearly this person must have no respect for the sanctity of the church. Her red, slinky, silk dress was more suited for a party, and to make it even worse, it was wrinkled. For the rest of the service, Rebecca was preoccupied with this example of the behavior of today's youth, who simply did not know how to conduct themselves appropriately. She was surprised when the movement of the congregation indicated that it was time for Communion; she had been completely distracted.

As the congregation began leaving the church, Rebecca had yet another surge of judgment. There, as bold as could be, was that young girl actually talking to the priest. Surely this person had no shame whatsoever. As Rebecca moved closer, she overheard the young woman sharing her experience with the priest. The night before, the young woman and her fiancé were on their way home from their engagement party. They were hit by a speeding motorist who ran a red light. The young woman had spent the night at the emergency room, praying that her fiancé would survive. After hours of waiting, she saw the doctor, who told her that her fiancé would have a full recovery. With overwhelming feelings of relief and gratitude, she knew that despite her weariness and the need to go home and shower and rest, she wanted to stop by her church and give thanks to God.

Rebecca listened and absorbed the information in silence. She could hear the words from Matthew 7:1 (NKJV), "Judge not, that you be not judged ... Why do you look at the speck that is in your brother's eye, but do not consider the plank in your own eye?" She raised her eyes and whispered, "Okay, God. I got the message."

Consider how much time Rebecca wasted with all that negative energy. Instead of being prayerful and grateful for blessings, Rebecca was embroiled in a cauldron of anger and blame. Her judgmental thoughts were like emotional cholesterol clogging the arteries of her soul. With more than five hundred references to "do not judge" in the Bible, can we come to a place of humility and leave the final judgment to God?

> Judging others is a heavy burden.
> —The Desert Fathers, fourth century

Being judgmental is learned behavior. There is a poignant song from the movie *South Pacific*, with these lyrics: "You've got to be taught before it's too late, before you are six, or seven or eight, to hate all the people your relatives hate, you've got to be carefully taught ..."

Prejudice is so pervasive that children can be cruel to other children who are different or have disabilities, because they learned these hateful attitudes. Fortunately, this can be unlearned and replaced with new learning.

Adapting an old saying, "Nonjudgmental actions speak louder than words," certainly rang true in the following situation. In March 1941, First Lady Eleanor Roosevelt hopped in the back of pilot C. Alfred "Chief" Anderson's plane at the Tuskegee Army Air Field in Alabama and went for a flight. This was not the simple act it would be today. This was a powerful message—because airman Anderson was black. Clearly, Mrs. Roosevelt had no energy to waste on prejudice (to prejudge).

The First Lady's visit marked the initiation of the US Army's African American pilot program and the activation of the first all–African American military aviation unit: the Ninety-Ninth Pursuit Squadron. Later named the Fighter Squadron, it became the first squadron of black pilots to fight in World War II in the skies over Pantelleria, an island near Sicily, on June 2, 1943.

A way to break the negativity of judging is to pause and recognize that everyone you meet has a story. When a judgmental thought comes up, stop, breathe, and go to curiosity to identify the source of that thought and arrive at a place of understanding. Accepting that there is always more going on behind the scenes in people's personal lives and having compassion for self and others will relieve you of the burden of judgment and restore your peace.

As you evolve, you can bypass judgment and go directly to compassion without any need to know the story. It is a process. At first, you get angry and judgmental when someone rudely cuts you off in traffic. At the next stage, someone cuts you off, and you get angry until you learn that he is rushing to the hospital to visit a loved one who is going into major surgery, and your anger and judgment dissolve. Finally, someone cuts you off, and you observe this nonjudgmentally and remain peaceful. Perhaps you recall times when you were the distracted driver who cut someone off.

You can also question your beliefs to uncover if there is any prejudice involved. Prejudice is one of the precursors to judgment that keeps you antagonistic, the us-versus-them attitude that keeps you focused on differences rather than similarities, with the need to feel superior. Knowing that prejudice is fueled by ignorance, you question the source and adjust your thinking to free you of this unhealthy burden.

The 1976 book *A Course in Miracles* states, "Today I shall judge nothing that occurs." Mother Teresa tells us that when you are judging, you are not loving, and when you are loving, you are not judging. Where there is judgment, there is no peace. When peace becomes your primary goal, you release the need to judge, and you let go of the fear of being judged.

Judgment can take place in even more subtle ways. When you see or hear someone else making judgments, it is easy to slip into that role of self-righteousness by thinking, *I can't believe that person is so judgmental; he really is an awful person.* In this situation, you have been seduced into judging another person, and possibly his behavior bothers you because it is a behavior that you want to change in yourself. I can remember my mother reciting this quote many times:

> There is so much good in the worst of us, and
> so much bad in the best of us, that it doesn't
> behoove any of us to speak ill of the rest of us.

Similar quotes have been attributed to several people, including Edward Wallis Hoch, James Truslow Adams, Robert Louis Stephenson, Edgar Cayce. Great minds think alike—right?

There is a fine line between judgment and assessment. There were times when I entertained certain thoughts and later chastised myself for being judgmental. This prompted an in-depth exploration, and I came to this understanding of the difference.

When you are judging, you label the behavior and then transfer the label to the person and see them as bad, irresponsible, or whatever judgment you made. When you are judging, you usually feel anxious, angry, critical, sarcastic, and unkind, and your body reacts accordingly. It is not possible to be peaceful when you are caught up in judgment, with the fierce need to be right.

With assessment, you observe the behavior of others and arrive at your own conclusion. Depending on the relationship, you might choose to share your observations, if the other person is open and receptive. You hope the feedback will be helpful, as intended.

It is difficult to avoid judgment in cases of violence or abuse. Yet, you do not have to judge or hate the person. You can pray, believing that "Whatever one sows, that will he also reap" (Galatians 6:7–8), which is also known as the law of cause and effect. You understand that justice will be served by a far more capable and potent judge, whether you get to see it or not. Better use of your energy is compassion for all. Without judgment, you hope that the perpetrator will be rehabilitated and transformed.

The effects of our actions may be postponed but they are never lost. There is an inevitable reward for good deeds and an inescapable punishment of bad. Meditate upon this truth, and seek always to earn good wages from Destiny.
—Wu Ming Fu

There is also the burden of self-judgment. Who could possibly judge us more severely than we judge ourselves? Who can be our harshest critic? This was the journey for Chuck …

During the years of the roller-coaster existence of living with his wife's alcoholism, he had supported her through multiple treatments and done everything he knew to do, and still her drinking continued. A loving, responsible woman when she was sober, she became this distant, surly stranger when she drank. His frustration built to the point at which he had difficulty engaging with her whether she was sober or impaired. He felt like a failure as a husband, because he had not been able to fix the problem. What was wrong with him that she chose alcohol over him?

He judged himself very sternly for every unkind thing he ever said and for every time he felt disconnected when she approached him during periods of abstinence. His self-judgment ignored the endurance it took to live with chronic alcoholism, broken promises, remorse, and regret, which engulfed them both. He found it hard to understand how she could be a loving wife and mother and yet go back to drinking when she knew how much it hurt him.

He eventually understood that instead of being stuck in self-judgment, judgment, and blame, he could accept that he was powerless over her drinking and that alcoholism was "cunning and baffling." He had to take responsibility for his behavior, learn about alcoholism as a family disease, and work on the necessary changes to stop feeling angry and hopeless most of the time. This required honest self-evaluation, introspection, and the strong desire to motivate personal changes.

The marriage ended, and over time Chuck let go of the pain, disappointment, judgment, and self–judgment to reopen his heart to new experiences. Healing the past empowered Chuck and his former wife to move along their separate paths and wish each other well.

> Break your heart no longer. Each time you judge
> yourself, you break your heart. You stop feeding
> on the love that is the wellspring of your vitality.
> Now the time has come, your time, to live, to
> celebrate and to see the goodness that you are.
> —Kirpal Venanji

Whatever you convey to the universe comes back to you. Judging others does not help anyone, least of all you. Choose instead to transmit good thoughts, words, emotions, and deeds that are essential for a better world. This sets into motion an unseen chain of effects, and eventually the vibratory energy returns to the original source like the swing of the pendulum. Children grasp the analogy of the boomerang: as you throw out the boomerang, it comes back to you. Thus, they understand the importance of throwing out the good thoughts and wishes you desire.

Key Points

- Breathe.
- Identify your judgmental thoughts and behaviors.
- Avoid stereotyping.
- Recognize the destructive nature of judgment.
- Understand the difference between assessment and judgment.
- Learn to reframe the situations that trigger your judgment (chapter 11).
- Validate yourself each time you choose peace over judgment.

When you acknowledge that judgment creates separation and division, destroys relationships, activates your ugly trait, and robs you of your peace, you can shed the burden of judgment. When you were a baby, you certainly didn't judge anyone by their appearance, and life was simple. Reclaim your peaceful, loving self by replacing judgment with curiosity and compassion.

CHAPTER 13

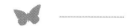

Replace Expectations with Hope

My hopes are not always realized, but I always hope.
—Ovid

Hope does not disappoint us. Hope sustains us because we know that life is a journey of hills, plateaus, and valleys. Expectations, on the other hand, set us up for disappointments. Often the invitation to let go of expectations elicits the response, "What about realistic expectations?" The clarifying question is, "What are realistic expectations, and for whom can we have these expectations?"

The logical answer is we can have expectations for ourselves, which we transform into goals to motivate action. Yet the expectations we have for ourselves can be self-defeating if we are driven by the need to be perfect, with an intense fear of failure. Expectations, by their very nature, require concrete results within the time frame we have prescribed, and when unmet, bring feelings such as frustration and resentment. A handy way to create a visual representation is to think about the *x* in expectations (get rid of them) and the *o* in hope, the shape of a lifesaver, to sustain us as we find our way.

To carry an expectation is to have an
appointment with disappointment.
—Vedic meditation students

103

Betty had spent most of her day doing several tasks with her daughter, and she was pleased that she had been able to help her daughter in this practical way. As they were parting, her daughter got out of the car, waved goodbye, and drove away. Betty's immediate thought was, *Well, is it asking too much to expect a simple thank you for everything we've done today?* as she fell back into that old feeling of being unappreciated. She took a conscious breath and remembered to hit her pause button. The acronym WAIT (chapter 3) came to mind, and Betty smiled and reminded herself that giving was a complete act of generosity, and any expression of gratitude was a bonus.

When they got together later that evening, Betty's daughter said to her, "Mom, I really want to thank you for everything you did today and tell you how grateful I am that you're there for me through this difficult time." Betty smiled as she gave her daughter a hug. Had she acted out on her unmet expectations earlier, she would have derailed this moment. This was so much more that the casual "thank you" that she would have received when her daughter exited the car. The moments of silence had served Betty well, as she used that time to process that first negative thought.

> I'm not in this world to live up to your expectations,
> and you're not in this world to live up to mine.
> —Bruce Lee

Sometimes there are unrealistic expectations. A couple who had never ventured beyond their small town was given a honeymoon package to an exotic island off the coast of South America. They were excited and very apprehensive. When they returned home, they expressed their disappointment and irritation. They had expected everyone to speak English, and they had not expected there to be all those "foreigners."

My happiness grows in direct proportion to my acceptance, and in inverse proportion to my expectations.
—Michael J. Fox

Perhaps one of the biggest triggers for expectations is holidays. Most years have 365 days; some have 366 days. Through some arbitrary process, we determined that certain of these days would be special, and we would call them holidays. If you harbored expectations regarding what others should do or give at these times, then the probability of being disappointed, sad, or angry was very high. In the recovering community, expectations have been described as "premeditated resentments." The Dalai Lama cautions that if there are no limits to your desires, you will not attain contentment.

There is a story of two young girls who grew up in different countries. Carla was the youngest of four children of her widowed mother. There was always food and shelter but never too much left over for extra things. Carla hoped she would have a gift or two under the Christmas tree. She knew the sacrifices her mother had to make to afford the gifts for the family.

Maggie, on the other hand, had parents who, although they could ill afford it, showered her with seemingly endless amount of gifts, overcompensating for their own childhood of scarcity. For Maggie, Christmas was an overwhelming array of gifts. She learned early in life that more was better, which meant high expectations and feelings of entitlement.

In adulthood, Maggie would plunge into debt every year to replicate the frenzy of gift giving that she had experienced with her own parents. She would expect her children to maintain that pitch of excitement throughout hours of tearing packages open. Maggie would dread the inevitable letdown when it was all over. The children would leave to play with their friends, and she would face months of repaying her credit cards. Eventually, Maggie learned the meaning of "less is more," and she subdued her impulsive spending in the hope of giving her children the new message of appreciation versus expectation.

> If all the year were playing holidays, to
> play would be as tedious as to work.
> —Hal in *King Henry IV*

It has been determined that overindulgence is the subtlest form of child abuse. This concept has become so widespread that there are workshops and seminars to address this problem. The more indulgent your parents were, or you are as a parent, the greater the potential for dissatisfaction later in life. If Christmas or other special holidays mean expectations of tons of gifts, the perfect family, food, drink, and limitless fun, then disappointment is almost guaranteed.

> I make myself rich by making my wants few.
> —David Henry Thoreau

Hope keeps you open to all possibilities and focused on the positive. When negative thoughts arise, you witness the discouragement and fear, gently let them go, and return to hope. When Melissa's husband lost his battle with cancer, the medical expenses left her in a very precarious financial situation. She took a course to equip her for a job and a path to becoming debt-free. Each week, she would purchase a lotto ticket, and whenever she felt really scared, she would hope that her troubles would be over when she had the winning ticket at the next drawing. Going from hopeless to hopeful was a shift in thinking. Twenty years later, she had not won the lotto yet, but this hope sustained her while she steadfastly made her way back to financial security.

> While I breathe, I hope.
> —South Carolina state motto

It's been said that there is only one hope that is futile, and that is hope for a different past. With hope, there is no time line or expiration date. Hope complements delayed gratification. A slogan to foster patience is "Time delay serves me." This concept is reinforced when things eventually unfold and you can look back at all the twists and turns along the path. With a better understanding of the whole picture, you see the value of hope. Hope opens the door for miracles to enter. A good acronym for hope is "heart open, please enter."

> Hope springs eternal.
> —Alexander Pope

Expectations can play a role in many situations. Caroline shared about her relationship with her parents. She always knew that her parents loved her and provided her and her siblings with a loving home. Yet she learned at an early age that they had their expectations of how she and her siblings would behave, who they were supposed to be friends with, the kind of careers they would pursue, even the kind of person they would marry. When her parents' expectations were not met, they made their disappointments known and lamented about where they had gone wrong.

Eventually, Caroline's parents realized that their expectations were damaging their relationships. They accepted that each of their children had the right to choose his or her own path. They discovered that when they let go of their expectations, they could enjoy their children's accomplishments. They hoped that their children would be happy, based on their children's definition of happiness, not theirs. Suffering begins with expectations and ends with acceptance.

> To expect something from another because it's our right
> is to court unhappiness. Others can and will only give
> what they are able, not what you desire they give.
> —Leo Buscaglia, *Love*

Ironically, expectations can take you to the other extreme. You ruminate on distressing thoughts such as *he/she will never change, nothing good ever happens to me, I always have bad luck, friends always let you down, my life will never get better.* Attempting to avoid disappointment, you anticipate not getting what you desire and experience some grim satisfaction from each unfortunate experience that justifies your bitterness.

> When nothing is sure, everything is possible.
> —Margaret Drabble

Hope sustains you as you navigate through challenging times. Choose to live each day open and receptive to all the good. Don't be limited by negative expectancy. Observe and remove barriers, such as unfounded doubts and fears, and keep the focus on the positive. Hope creates the space for abundance to flow in.

> Loss, a worry, an illness, a dream, no matter how deep
> your hurt or how high your aspirations, do yourself a
> favor and pause as least once per day to place your hands
> over your heart and say aloud "Hope lives here."
> —Sandra King

Key Points

- Breathe.
- Recognize how expectations set you up for disappointment and frustration.
- See challenges as part of the journey.
- Visualize what you desire and allow hope to sustain you along the way.
- Learn to be content in uncertainty.
- Be grateful and encouraged by every blessing.

There is a significant correlation between expectations and disappointments. The more expectations you have, especially expectations of other people, the greater potential for disappointments. Hope keeps you aligned with the intention, free of attachment to the outcome. Hope is strengthened by acceptance. Seek to be encouraged, secure in the knowledge that things will work out exactly as they were meant to, enhanced by the sustaining power of hope and faith.

CHAPTER 14

Don't Worry. It Doesn't Help.

"What—Me Worry?"
—The fictional mascot, Alfred E. Newman, a gap-toothed,
freckled kid who never worries

Everyone experiences the emotional reaction of worrying about a threat in the uncertain future. You can't escape issues that can activate this emotion. You can learn how to take control of worrying rather than have worrying take control of your mind.

Worry thoughts can strike at any time. For example, the sleepless night before you make your presentation to hundreds of participants at a conference, you become terrified by all the things that could go wrong, despite knowing that you are fully prepared and confident. Fear is often a shadow without substance. The next day, your presentation goes well, and you determine that you have to change your consciousness about worry. You commit to finding healthy alternatives.

Habitual worrying has harmful side effects—irritability, fatigue, difficulty concentrating, restlessness, and a host of health issues. At times, worry can feel unbearable.

Worry is a misuse of the imagination.
—Dan Zadra

Worry can also evolve from unresolved childhood issues, such as embarrassment, abandonment, and tragedy. You can do the therapeutic work to connect today's feelings to similar feelings from the past, to understand, resolve, and release the source of your debilitating thoughts. Thus you become empowered to determine which worries alert you to pay attention and which are simply repetitive, exhausting, and unnecessary.

> I've had a lot of worries in my life,
> most of which never happened.
> —Mark Twain

The following story shows the importance of shifting the focus away from worry.

When Lorna learned that her son, George, was using drugs, she lived in a constant state of fear. She ruminated about "what if" and "why." She would say repeatedly to George, "It's impossible not to worry. I'm your mother. What if you were in a car accident or pulled over by the police? What if you were arrested and got a record and could not be accepted by private colleges? Why do you make me worry all the time? If you really loved me, you would stop this crazy behavior that is making me sick with worry." Lorna's anxiety about her son's behavior became toxic to their relationship and spilled over to the family dynamic with her husband and daughter. Their home environment was often filled with tension.

When George was ready to seek help, he went to a treatment center, and the family participated. Through the education and counseling, they learned about the complexity of addiction, codependency, and the coping skills to sustain them through the recovery process. Interestingly, they discovered how this changed the way they approached other life challenges. For example, they didn't have to be stuck in worry; they could move on to awareness, concern, patience, acceptance, and hope.

One day, George called to share with Lorna that he was having a particularly bad day. He was fighting the cravings to use drugs. She listened and felt the usual sharp twinge of fear. He asked her please not to worry, that he knew that he had to call his sponsor and go to a meeting to get through this hard time. Lorna breathed and said a prayer. Then she tackled all the tasks she had scheduled for the day. Around six o'clock, George called her again to let her know that he was feeling much better. He thanked her for listening and always being there for him. He added, "I must say you've really changed. In the past, you would have called me every half an hour, and I would have felt guilty for burdening you with my problem. Instead, you allowed me to talk about my cravings while you took the time to listen. I guess we're both learning."

Lorna hung up the phone and considered what George had said. In the past, just hearing about cravings could generate negative projections of drastic consequences. By changing her thinking, she had avoided unnecessary suffering. She knew that *caring was not the same as worrying*, and you can learn as much from mistakes as from accomplishments, perhaps more. She thought about the old proverb, "Don't cross the bridge until you come to it." Furthermore, "Don't build bridges over rivers that don't exist." She recognized the power of acceptance, prayer, and gratitude for ongoing recovery. Let your "what if" become "what if something positive."

Another situation with Marina and her son illustrates the futility of worrying. Marina would wait up and struggle with fear until all hours of the night or early morning until her son came home. She would sometimes hide in the shadows so her son would not see her. Once she knew he was safely home, she would breathe a sigh of relief and finally go to bed.

One evening, Marina got the call every parent dreads. The police officer at the other end of the phone told her that her son was being airlifted to Jackson Memorial Hospital Trauma Center after having been struck by a car while he was Rollerblading. How paradoxical that tragedy had not struck at two or three o'clock in the morning at the height of her stressful projections but rather on an ordinary evening! This was not even one of the many scenarios that she had imagined night after night.

That night, Marina felt a stoic calmness as she and her husband got ready to make their way to the trauma center. She heard again the words of the officer, "Please drive carefully." In this real emergency, she had to be clearheaded and focused to provide the support her son needed. Clearly, worrying in advance had been completely useless.

> Worrying does not take away tomorrow's
> troubles; it takes away today's peace.
> —Randy Armstrong

Two ways to relate to a problem are worry or make a plan. With worry, you generally ruminate and agonize about an indefinite future. Each problem reinforces the fear that things will only get worse. Your worries inundate most of your conversations and wear down friends and family.

Making a plan, on the other hand, places the focus on the solution. You review the situation to see if there is anything you can do to contribute to the solution. You replace worry with calming alternatives like prayer or meditation and invite feedback from others who overcame similar challenges. This brings more clarity and encouragement.

Your life experience changes when you discover that

letting go of worry is the act of shifting your focus to what you want and away from what you fear. When the storm has passed, you can validate yourself for avoiding the pitfalls of this debilitating emotion by taking each day as it comes.

> Remember, today is the tomorrow
> you worried about yesterday.
> —Dale Carnegie

"Also," John contributed to the group discussion, "today can be the tomorrow you prayed for yesterday."

The following story illustrates how to circumvent worrying about a practical issue by looking for a possible solution.

Judith checked her work schedule and discovered that despite her attempts to set healthy boundaries, the scheduler had assigned her an excessive number of appointments for one day. She faced a choice. She could ruminate and complain about this injustice for the next few weeks, feeling increasing dread as the date approached, or she could look for another option.

With further investigation, she discovered that the scheduler had made a mistake, and this was not a regular workday for her. She had been flexible in adjusting her days around their needs, and she had a choice to go into work that day or not. She advised the scheduler well in advance that she would be away at that time. She used this time as a "health day" to visit her family. Rather than worry and feel victimized, she redirected her energy to explore alternatives. Thus, she saved herself needless anguish.

> That the birds of worry fly above your head,
> this you cannot change. But that they build their
> nests in your hair, this you can prevent.
> —Chinese proverb

In the movie *Bridge of Spies*, Tom Hanks plays James Donovan, the attorney who defended a Russian spy and then negotiated his exchange for an American pilot held by the Soviet Union, during the height of the Cold War. There is a scene when James Donovan looks at the Russian spy, puzzled at the man's calm demeanor when he knows the severe ramifications he is facing. Donovan says, "I have a mandate to serve you. Everyone else seems to have an interest in sending you to the electric chair." After a brief pause, Donovan continues, "You don't seem alarmed." The spy responds, "Would it help?" You can use these logical words to adopt a similar attitude when your mind wants to propel you into another useless worry cycle. You can reflect on a refrain from that old Doris Day song, "Que sera, sera, whatever will be will be, the future's not ours to see, que sera, sera, what will be, will be."

Key Points

- Breathe.
- Witness the worry thoughts and the physical effects.
- Determine if there is anything you need to do in that moment.
- Harness that energy and apply it to appropriate action.
- Identify any similarity with feelings from the past and commit to addressing and resolving them.
- If there is nothing to do in the moment, relax and replace worry with prayer, meditation, and so on.
- Be gentle as you mindfully release all worry thoughts.
- Go from fear to flow.
- Recite positive affirmations to maintain your freedom.

If you pray, why worry? If you worry, why pray?
—Adapted from Philippians 4:6

When you accept the futility of worry and redirect your energy to healthy alternatives, you appreciate each new day. Your loved ones will enjoy your caring without the burden of your worry. Perhaps you'll hum along with the song "Don't Worry, Be Happy."

Chapter 15

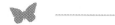

Let Go of the Need to Control Others

When you try to control everything, you enjoy nothing.
—Unknown

Controlling behaviors often arise from the desire to get others to think and act the way you want. This need to control may come from a caring place; for example, when you see your loved ones going in the wrong direction, and you want desperately to spare them the inevitable consequences. Your communication is filled with shoulds, and you hijack conversations to interject your advice.

A distressed mother named Bella said, "I must control you, because when you fail, I fail, and then I have to make it right." Her overinvolvement meant that she suffered while her son dismissed the repercussions of his poor choices. Her anxiety was fueled by the belief that there must be some way for her to make her son change.

The parents' role is challenging. There are many situations in which a child depends on the protection of the parents and, in fact, might not survive without this protection. Yet the belief that parents have control over all situations increases the vulnerability to self-blame and disappointment. Any parent who has experienced unforeseen tragedy with a child can attest to having to let go of the fantasized ability to protect the ones you love. The distress from lack of control needs to be replaced with acceptance and faith.

A parent's role is to give their children roots and then one day to give them wings. A disciplined process of transferring responsibility empowers the child to build resilience and self-reliance. When the goal becomes to let go of control, what do you do? You do your part and let go of attachment to the outcome. Instead of trying to control and take over, you contribute to the process and respect the other person's ability to find the way. Thus, the real challenge is to determine what will be helpful. Sometimes the line between helping and controlling can be confusing. So, good questions to ask yourself are "Will this help the person grow, or will my action simply remove the consequence and delay accountability?" and "Is this a short-term solution to a long-term problem to rescue the person and relieve my anxiety?"

Enabling is disabling when it impedes growth. There may be times, for instance, when you are financially able to pay off someone's debts. You ask yourself the age-old question, "Just because I can, does that mean I should?" Sometimes only when you are no longer able to fix it does the other person get the opportunity to face the repercussions, take responsibility, and grow. The longer the enabling continues, the harder it will be for the person to handle the escalating consequences. It can be painful to let go, even after you understand that it is the right thing to do. Love keeps you connected, free of the need to control.

Discovering the difference between sympathy, empathy, and compassion can bring a shift in perception. Sympathy implies that you feel sorry for those "poor" people, and this can contribute to their self-pity, victimhood, and low self-worth. Empathy is identifying with and mirroring the other's feelings. There is a line from a meditation that states, "Help me find compassion without empathy overwhelming me." This captures the need to be aware of the intense feelings from taking on the weight of the other person's experience. Excessive emotional empathy can negatively impact your health. Compassion understands and validates their struggle and emotions, and it salutes their hope and courage to overcome the challenges. Thus, sympathy can be disempowering (fostering helplessness), empathy is relating to the challenge (supportive), and compassion is empowering (supporting self-reliance).

> If passion drives you, let reason hold the reins.
> —Benjamin Franklin

There are times when you need to step in. If your loved one becomes too impaired to make crucial decisions, as in the case of people who struggle with addiction or alcoholism, get professional help. Provide support and replace judgment with patience and understanding.

This is an example of knowing when to take action. Sally was in family group with her father, Roger. She had been in treatment for two months, with minimal contact with her father. She indicated to the group therapist that she was ready to share. She took a deep breath. She started by thanking her father for taking the risk of having her hate him by getting the Marchman Act to mandate her to treatment. She had been intensely angry with him at the beginning, believing that everyone blamed her for being a bad person and destroying the family. Now she had an understanding of addiction and the suffering it caused. She expressed her gratitude for the life in recovery that was now possible with a commitment—one day at a time—to sobriety and growth.

Roger took a moment to arrange his thoughts. He said that words could not express his gratitude for Beth's change of heart and how much he had learned by participating in the program. He added that he would be by her side on her new journey. Here was a case where Roger could only do his part of getting Sally to treatment, and the rest was up to her. He understood that controlling behavior disrupts human connection. He would strengthen their relationship by adhering to the guidelines for the recovering family. He would love her unconditionally and strive to trust the process.

Be patient, until the miracle happens.

Another recovery story shows the value of patience. Patrick's brother struggled with chronic alcoholism. Several times, his brother survived near-death experiences with the help of the urgent responses to 911 emergency calls. Patrick would sometimes use humor to disguise his apprehension that his brother might not survive the next relapse. He would say with a sad chuckle that he was getting to know the first names of the EMT technicians. When fear threatened to overwhelm Patrick, he relied on the Serenity Prayer.

God, grant me the Serenity to accept the things
I cannot change, courage to change the things I
can, and wisdom to know the difference.
—Reinhold Niebuhr

Through the Serenity Prayer, Patrick accepted that, despite all his efforts, he could not control his brother's drinking and consequences. With the "wisdom to know the difference," he would do what was helpful and let go of the rest. Acceptance gave him the loving detachment that kept him from plunging into resignation and giving up in despair. He learned the difference between stepping aside (to allow his brother to take responsibility) versus walking away (abandonment). Patrick continued to do everything he could to support his brother, including prayer. He was fortified by the saying, "When fear knocks on the door, open it with faith."

Patrick recognized that this was his brother's journey. Like Humpty Dumpty in the nursery rhyme by Mother Goose, "Humpty Dumpty sat on a wall, Humpty Dumpty had a great fall; all the king's horses and all the king's men, couldn't put Humpty together again," only Patrick's brother could put himself back together again. Surrender and openness to guidance would make this possible. When impatience, frustration, and despair threatened his peace, Patrick used the Serenity Prayer to stabilize and return to acceptance and hope. He also recited the phrase "Patience gains all things," which he related to his brother's changes as well as his own.

One day, the miracle happened. His brother broke through denial, asked for help, and began the journey to recovery. Patrick felt great relief after all the years of hoping and trusting the process. Patrick was fully aware that recovery was not guaranteed, and he was grateful every day that his brother embraced a concrete recovery program.

The next story shows another type of situation that cannot be controlled. Members of an annual ski group were checking in for their return flight home. They were told that the flight would be delayed. One passenger, Harry, went into a tirade at the check-in counter about the value of his time and the great inconvenience the delay would cause. He stormed over to the group leader and demanded, "Well, what are you going to do about this?"

Beau, the group leader, was calmly doing some work on his laptop computer. He looked up and said, "I have learned that a delayed flight results from one of three issues: problems with the weather, the equipment, or the pilot. If any one or more of these is the problem, I feel much safer here on the ground. I'd suggest that you find a peaceful way to pass the time." Beau hoped that Harry realized the only thing he could control was his attitude.

You can't stop the waves, but you can learn to surf.
—Jon Kabat-Zinn

Jill's story illustrates the frustration that can arise from others not following your helpful advice. This was Jill's experience with her good friend Hilde. Despite Jill's encouragement, supported by research articles and simple alternatives, Hilde would not make changes to provide a healthy diet for her child. Yet Hilde would complain about his allergies and negative behaviors, which in turn caused all sorts of stress for her. Hilde always had multiple excuses to resist Jill's recommendations, and Jill's distress came from seeing this child suffer needlessly.

One day, a mutual friend gave Jill something to consider the next time she was tempted to give Hilde advice. "Ask yourself, is this something I haven't said before? Is there something new to say?" Jill smiled and acknowledged her friend's wisdom. She actually felt relief at not having to engage in the old "Why don't you? Yes, but ..." game that had been so exhausting for her. She reflected on the many conservations when she would make a suggestion like, "Would you consider cutting back on the sugary drinks?" and Hilde would immediately reply, "Yes, but you know how much he looks forward to his chocolate at night." And if Jill continued, "What about the daytime drinks?" Hilde would respond, "Yes, but you know I already bought a case of his favorite drink."

Jill realized that her role was to set a good example of diet and nutrition when they were together, and the child could learn to make his own healthy choices as he matured. Jill also learned the technique, when making a suggestion, to end with "or not." When Jill invited Hilde to try something new, *or not*, it removed the option of resistance, because Hilde would be complying either way. This also helped Jill let go of attachment to the outcome and subsequent frustration.

Preach the gospel. When necessary, use words.
—Attributed to St. Francis of Assisi

Rick said he remembered hearing this comment, "If it's raining and your roof is leaking, you can either fix your roof or change the weather." He recounted all the times his anxiety had come from not being able to fix someone or something. Sometimes there can be an intense sense of urgency when you strongly disapprove of another person's actions and feel the desperate need to change them.

Control can wear a disguise in the form of questions. If you watched the TV series *Columbo*, you will remember his famous line: "Just one more thing." Columbo would have endless questions until the villain was worn down and apprehended.

If you have ever engaged in inflicting a barrage of questions on your loved one, chances are you were told that it felt suffocating or overwhelming by the resentful recipient. Since this is the opposite of what you intended, recognize the destructive nature of this way of communicating. When your approach begins to feel like interrogation, you can catch it and lighten up with the code word "Columbo."

Letting go of control means you accept that you are powerless over certain things, not to be confused with helpless. Helpless and hopeless often go together, feeling that nothing will ever get better. This leads to resignation and feeling defeated. Powerless, on the other hand, comes from knowing what is beyond your control. Acceptance of your powerlessness does not mean that you condone the behavior, simply that you cannot control it. You determine what actions will contribute to the solution, without needing to take the credit or the blame for the outcome.

Sometimes surrender means giving up trying to understand and becoming comfortable with not knowing.
—Eckhart Tolle

Feeling uncomfortable often triggers the need to control. You can learn to tolerate this feeling and become comfortable with discomfort. With this internal change, you process negative thoughts differently and gently bid them go. Breathe and remember to *hold the vision* and *trust the process*.

This brings to mind a cute cartoon about two friends who go to see a psychologist. When asked what brought them to therapy, this was the response: "Hi, my friend and I aren't getting along, and I was hoping you could help us by blaming him for everything and making him change." The psychologist replied, "I'm afraid that's not how therapy works." The friend spoke again: "Perhaps you're not a good fit for us."

It seems appropriate to wind down this chapter with the following classic anecdote. The original of the story is attributed to Frank Koch, a naval officer. One night, the lookout on the bridge suddenly shouted, "Captain! A light bearing on the starboard bow."

"Is it stationary or moving astern?" the captain asked. The lookout replied that it was stationary. This meant the battleship was on a dangerous collision course with the other ship. The captain immediately ordered his signalman to signal to the ship: "We are on a collision course. I advise you to change course twenty degrees east."

Back came a response from the other ship: "You change course twenty degrees west."

Agitated by the arrogance of the response, the captain asked his signalman to shoot out another message: "I am a captain. You change course twenty degrees east."

Back came the second response: "I am a second-class seaman. You had still better change course twenty degrees west."

The captain was furious this time! He shouted to the signalman to send back a final message: "I am a battleship. Change course twenty degrees east right now!"

Back came the flashing response: "I am a lighthouse." The captain duly changed course.

This experience certainly gave the captain an opportunity to reevaluate his sense of self-importance. Being arrogant or being calm and collected had no bearing on the facts. Curiosity and flexibility will help you identify what represents the battleship versus the lighthouse in your own life, to determine what you can or cannot control or change. With this understanding, you are open to all possibilities and ready to take appropriate action or simply let go.

At the end of a discussion, John gave this feedback: "One of the scariest lessons I have learned is that sometimes there is nothing I can do. One of the most beautiful lessons I have learned is that most of the time I don't have to, and it is better if I don't."

Fear can trigger you to fall back into futile attempts to control. Concern, on the other hand, is being aware without going to despair. Explore situations from a broader perspective. Be grateful for the positive. Direct your energy to change what you can and accept that there are some things that you cannot control. Acceptance fosters serenity.

Key Points

- Breathe.
- Explore the situation to identify options.
- Apply the Serenity Prayer.
- Make a plan of action for things within your control.
- Accept your powerlessness over things you cannot control.
- Use your imagination to visualize a positive outcome.
- Know that there is opportunity in adversity.
- Learn the lesson embedded in the event.
- Let love, not fear, guide your decisions.

Realize how few things you can control and resign as master of the universe. Identify your part, take appropriate action, and let go of the rest. Use your imagination to visualize what you want, rather than letting fear create what you do not want. Reinforce your resilience. Be patient. Look for miracles.

CHAPTER 16

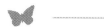

Practice Positive, Compassionate Confrontation

> The goal of compassionate confrontation is to generate mutual understanding before taking action.
> —Unknown

Confrontation is often seen as hostility between opposing parties. This can be a barrier to understanding the importance of compassionate confrontation. The above quote expresses the goal of this chapter, to present positive, compassionate confrontation as a building block for healthy relationships.

Many people declare that they hate confrontation and avoid it at all costs. They eventually accumulate a buildup of unexplored, unexpressed resentments, and the proverbial last straw sets off an explosion. At this point, the bottled-up pain erupts as hurtful anger. In the aftermath, the anger recedes into a smoldering pit without any resolution. The cycle starts over.

> If nothing changes, nothing changes.
> —Unknown

Positive confrontation is a way to create clarity and identify options. A relationship where confrontation is avoided will probably mean little or no expression of feelings, misunderstood feelings, and a corresponding lack of trust and closeness. The issue is not whether to confront or not but rather how and when to confront. Effective confrontation needs to take place within certain parameters.

Confrontation that comes from a place of fear can attract defensiveness and disrupt the communication. Confronting in anger will render the confrontation ineffective and could make the problem worse. You must take the time to move from fear to love to be able to operate from a peaceful place, clearly understanding the intention. "What is my motive?" is a good question to ask yourself. "Do I want to address an unresolved issue from the past? Is this a concern about current behaviors?"

Compassionate confrontation does not mean that the other person will change immediately, as the following story shows. When Benny met Isabel, he was attracted to her outgoing personality. She was flirtatious, and she liked when people referred to her as sexy. He was fascinated by her Hispanic culture, and he thought he might take Spanish lessons to bridge the gap with her family and friends. He felt he was the envy of every man when she was on his arm. They married after a short courtship.

Several years later, his perception changed. He felt jealous and insecure when she received too much attention. He decided to confront her about his discomfort. Isabel listened quietly. She told him that it was interesting that he now wanted her to change the things that had attracted him to her in the first place. If he felt that way now, perhaps he should have stayed with his shy ex-wife, who dressed very modestly.

In this example, Benny expressed his concerns, and his wife expressed her feelings. If Benny demanded that Isabel change, this would not be confronting; this would be an attempt to control. His options were to change his perception for his peace of mind, explore the possibility of compromise, continue suffering, or end the relationship.

Confront the behaviors, not the person. Talk about the behaviors you observed, what you felt, and your concerns about the potential consequences. This could occur, for example, if you suspected that your loved one was regressing to old addictive conduct. The conversation might go like this. "I am grateful for all the positive changes you have been making and your accomplishments of getting a job and rebuilding your life. I am concerned because I am observing some of the behaviors that were present when you were abusing drugs. You come home late and go straight to your room. Last night, you left on all the lights in the kitchen, there was food left out on the counter, and the front door was unlocked, and you seem irritated most of the time. When you were enthusiastic about your recovery, you were peaceful, responsible, and communicative. I want to remind you that I am here for you, and your recovery is our greatest gift. Can we talk about it?" In this way, you have clearly stated what you have seen, and you have not attacked the person with accusations and threats.

There can be any number of responses. Be prepared to witness the reaction and recognize that this is the other person's way of dealing with what you said. You are simply providing information, and the outcome is not up to you. Often, this approach will open a dialogue and refocus on the solution. Once you have said what you needed to say, you simply let go, unless this is an extreme situation that requires further appropriate action. It is important to determine whether this is about control, fueled by a sense of urgency, and this can be clarified by inviting feedback from a supportive person who understands the dynamic.

This story shows how two sisters handled confrontation in adulthood. The older sister, Mary, was quiet and reserved and generally had very little to say. She was the "good" child who studied hard and never got involved in her parents' arguments. The younger sister, Lilly, was very outgoing, often getting into trouble, and her low performance in school was always compared to her sister, Mary's, excellent grades. The older sister would shudder when she saw the severe punishments Lilly received, which did not seem to deter her acting-out behaviors. In fact, Lilly would not even flinch when she was beaten, and she would smile just to show that it did not hurt. As they grew older, the gap between them widened, to the point where Mary's secretary would screen her calls so that Mary could avoid speaking with Lilly.

Years later, Lilly sought out therapy to make some sense of her chaotic life. As she got in touch with the soul behind her mask, she began to see herself as the misunderstood child who hid behind the wall of indifference. She found the courage to invite her sister, Mary, to join her in an individual family session. Mary agreed to meet with the therapist first, to overcome her reluctance to being exposed to her sister's "craziness." After the meeting, Mary agreed to the joint session.

Guidelines were established at the beginning, with the understanding that if at any time it became too uncomfortable, the session could be halted and if necessary rescheduled. Lilly agreed to listen as Mary confronted her with all the pent-up feelings of the past: stories of the perceived disrespect, hurtful behaviors, and insensitivity. Lilly listened quietly as the tears gently began to trickle down her cheeks. The room became really quiet after Mary ended, and she seemed exhausted and relieved as she allowed her tears to flow. Lilly sobbed as she surrendered to years of blocked feelings, years of coping by eating to shut down any emotions, and the self-loathing as she saw herself becoming lost in her own body.

In the silence, Mary and Lily began to experience the

sensation of heavy weights being lifted. Lilly spoke haltingly. "I never had any idea that I caused you so much pain. I was busy hiding my own feelings of worthlessness and rejection, pretending not to care, knowing that everyone saw me as a big disappointment when compared to you. I felt as if everyone loved you and hated me. When I heard you so cautiously describe all my hateful behaviors, I felt such remorse, and I hope we still have time to heal our relationship."

During the sessions that followed, each was able to explore unresolved issues, gain clarity, seek and give forgiveness, and let go of the burden of resentment that they had carried all those years. Lilly said, "I can't tell you how wonderful it was that first time that Mary took my phone call." Mary replied, "I can't tell you how great it is to look forward to her calls."

It took courage to walk through the fear and confront the issues in a descriptive, nonjudgmental way, with the clear intention of finding peace and building a loving relationship. In a safe setting with good intentions, the process that they had dreaded opened the path to healing and connection. Compassionate confrontation made this possible. Not every situation will be resolved this way, but willingness to do your part is the first step.

Another example was Daisy's situation at work. Her associate, Jonah, would come to her office and slide the items on her desk over to make room to sit on the corner of her desk. Daisy really liked Jonah but found his behavior very annoying. Her chest would tighten up the minute Jonah entered her office, and this would be distracting during their conversation. She would deliberately put all the items back in place as soon as he left her office. She never said anything to Jonah, and this anxiety kept building to the point that it began to interfere with their friendship. Finally, Daisy was coached to share her feelings with Jonah. She followed the steps: she validated his friendship, identified the behavior in a descriptive, nonjudgmental way, and asked if he would sit in the chair instead. Jonah was a little defensive at first and suggested that they talk later.

After Daisy had the time to clear the air with Jonah, their heartfelt conversation revealed other underlying issues. Strengthened by this insight, Daisy went on to confront other challenging situations. If the other person's behavior did not change, she did not have to continue to be annoyed. She was free to accept it or avoid it.

Confronting can be a way to clarify why a husband never has the time to participate in social events with his wife. The approach could be, "I hear you saying that you want to come to the party with me, but then I also hear you telling me how pressed for time you are with all that you need to accomplish. This confuses me, and I am wondering what you really want to do." Here again, you would need to be able to be okay with the other person's response, having invited him to be honest. Of course, if he never wants to come to the party and always wants to work instead, then you would be dealing with a deeper issue, which would be very important to address.

Your emotional state plays a vital role in confronting an issue. In the recovering community, they talk about HALT. I expanded this by adding an S. This acronym stands for hungry, angry, lonely, tired, sick/scared. The recommendation is that you do not discuss anything important when you are in one or more of these states, because you will not be in a centered and grounded place to communicate your concerns.

If you are hungry, have something to eat.

If you are angry, take a deep breath, go for a walk, exercise, journal, or talk it over with a trusted friend, to come to a better understanding of the source of your anger.

If you are feeling lonely, remember that loneliness is a door that only opens from the inside. Expand your support system with kindred spirits who can be available for a phone call or a movie, rather than rely solely on one person to always be there.

If you are tired, get some rest. How many times have you misunderstood or been misunderstood simply because you were tired and irritable?

Finally, being sick or scared brings a greater feeling of vulnerability, and you can project all the things you do not want.

With this helpful acronym, you can slow down and consider the impact of your words. Approaching an issue in writing gives you the opportunity to reread it later from the perspective of the recipient. This is good to keep in mind when you are triggered to hit that reply button without taking the time to think it through. Sending the email to yourself and reading it when you have calmed down will give you better control of your response. This has been found to avert many potentially damaging situations. If you believe that you need anger or fear to propel you to get the pent-up words out, the other person may feel attacked, and the message will be lost.

Following a process will guide you to confront appropriately, free of any expectations. You identify and explore the issue to determine what you are thinking and feeling. When the feelings range from hurt or disappointment to anger and perhaps rage, you have to stabilize your thoughts. You take those three conscious breaths and move into the role of the witness and get in touch with your intention. Determine what you hope to accomplish with this conversation. If you are angry and simply want to vent, this can be done in a positive way to create the clarity necessary for compassionate confrontation. You can also journal these feelings and then tear up the paperwork and throw it away. If you have a support network of people you trust, you can share these thoughts and feelings with them. You ask yourself, "What would love do here?"

When you are prepared, you ask permission to give feedback. You choose your words wisely, and you allow the recipient to understand or dismiss your confrontation. You take a risk by being open and honest, not hurtful, because you care about the other person's well-being and your peace. A caution is to be prepared to lose the friendship if the other person shuts down. You hope for a positive result and accept whatever unfolds.

> I have several times made a poor choice by
> avoiding a necessary confrontation.
> —John Cleese

Confronting can be a prelude to boundaries, the topic of the next chapter. Annie's story is a good example of this. Annie had been enduring a distressing relationship with her son. She was intensely focused on his behaviors. She would resentfully pick up the clutter he left lying around their home—shoes, cups, glasses, bottles, and so on—and clean up the mess he left in the guest bathroom. If he was in a bad mood, he would be reactive and rude to her, and later feel alternating shame and anger. At times, she was fearful to even ask him a question. In sharing this with her support group, she realized that his intimidating behavior aroused similar feelings from her childhood with abusive parents.

One day she knew that she could not put off the conversation any longer. She validated his positive qualities, expressed her unconditional love, and compassionately confronted his disrespectful attitude toward her. She gently and firmly made it clear that he was welcome to visit only when he could be respectful in word and deed. She asked if there was anything she could do differently.

He explained how smothered he felt because of her intense attachment to his every action. He gave her an example and asked if she could stop being a helicopter mom. He added that he felt like a bully when she tolerated his aggression. Having confronted his behaviors and established a boundary, she knew it was time to let go. When she changed her debilitating question "Why is this happening *to me?*" to curiosity "Why is this happening?" she took ownership of her role in the disturbing relationship. She redirected her attention to personal change, self-care, and inner peace.

When communicating your wishes, you can apply the assertive model. Rather than expecting the other person to know what you want, you express your desire clearly and openly. Here is the communication model that was developed for assertive communication, the acronym DESC:

D—*describe* the behavior or request; identify the behavior in a descriptive, nonjudgmental manner.

E—*express* the feeling you are experiencing using "I statements" (when this happens, I feel ...).

S—*state* the need or want that you have (I would appreciate if you would ...).

C—*consequences*: explain what will be the positive outcome for you and for the other person, cognizant that you might not get the result you hope for (all that I will ask is what you are able to give).

When you are able to share your feelings and requests from a place of love, then fear or anger will not take over the conversation. Motivated by the intention of creating clarity, connection, and respect, you will caringly confront any issue in a descriptive, nonjudgmental way, without blame or attachment to a specific outcome. You are then free to let go, observe how things unfold, and determine if there is anything else you need to do.

Prepare by having these guidelines in place:

- Choose a safe place to have the meeting.

- Be sure that there is enough time to explore the issue and agree on the time allotted.
- Avoid times like bedtime or during meals.
- Remember HALTS—not when you are hungry, angry, lonely, tired, sick, or scared—or anyone has been drinking.

After establishing the above, you are ready to practice compassionate confrontation.

Key Points

- Breathe.
- Be peaceful and watch your tone. This will keep everyone listening and will help you get your point across.
- Breathe and relax to be able to respond, not react or attack.
- Begin with positive comments. Focusing on the things that are going right will illustrate that the request for change is intended to make things even better.
- Present the issues in a kind and considerate way. "I was wondering if we could discuss ..." Avoid the word "but."
- Ask the "confrontee" his or her thoughts and try to reach an agreement.
- Remember the requested change may not occur with the first try, or perhaps ever. Keep in mind that your efforts are part of your *gift* to that person, which can be used as desired.
- It is helpful to organize and write down your thoughts. This will help you keep it simple and ensure that your words are aligned with the intention. This also makes

it possible for you to reflect on what it would feel like to be on the receiving end of the confrontation.

- End the conversation on a positive note.

Positive, compassionate confrontation makes it possible for you to respectfully and safely explore differences and clarify issues. You stabilize your thoughts and feelings and share them. When you are confronting or being confronted, you do not engage in hostile confrontation. You wonder how the conversation will evolve. The intention is to make things better by increasing the understanding that strengthens relationships. You strive to move away from confusion and misunderstanding, and you accept the value of cooperation and compromise.

CHAPTER 17

Establish Clear, Healthy Boundaries

> Personal boundaries are guidelines or limits that a person
> creates to identify reasonable, safe and permissible ways
> for other people to behave towards them, and how
> they will respond when someone passes those limits.
> —Wikipedia

The simple way to think about boundaries is to reflect on the boundaries between countries. A driving vacation through Europe will take you across many boundaries, and you learn about the culture, food, language, and history of each country—how countries are similar or different. Boundaries between people are based on an understanding of beliefs and values. When you know what is important to you, you have the opportunity to explore areas of similarity or diversity. Boundaries are for self-protection.

The world today seems to be shrinking as people from many parts of the world find themselves suddenly trying to coexist. Without compassionate understanding, unnecessary conflict often arises. Boundaries are essential for healthy relationships with family, friends, colleagues, and others. Boundaries are about self-care and being considerate.

Without clear boundaries, there can be assumptions and expectations, which can lead to resentment, perceived disrespect, and dissatisfaction. Consider the situation with Richard and Aly …

Richard was the only child of wealthy parents who had very busy lives, and they gave Richard all the material things he could desire but very little of their time. They made it clear what was expected of him and the life that he was being prepared for. Aly, on the other hand, came from a large family. They were very involved with one another, and there was not much privacy.

There were several misunderstandings, as Richard had a clear definition of what was his, and Aly was used to sharing, often without even asking first. When their increasing arguments threatened to undermine their relationship, they had to learn about healthy boundaries and how to honor these boundaries to create the comfort they desired.

Among other things, they gained a deeper awareness of their cultural and historical differences. Richard's British heritage with its stiff-upper-lip philosophy was in stark contrast to Aly's Italian heritage, filled with affection and boisterous behaviors. They learned that boundaries are not designed to change the other person but rather to create safety and respect.

Boundaries give both people the opportunity to honor themselves and attend to their needs. It takes time and reflection to know your values and priorities, as these guide your actions. Boundaries also are individual, and you have to come to terms with which issues you are willing to compromise on and which issues are deal breakers. Otherwise, there remains a constant area of discord, with each expecting the other to change, keeping the focus on what is not working, thereby creating unnecessary suffering.

With time and effort, Richard and Aly learned to overcome the initial resistance that can occur while making life changes. With open communication, they could explore feelings, negotiate their differences, and meet somewhere in the middle. The best outcome is where each can take the best from the other, with alternating roles of student and teacher, growing individually and as a couple. Boundaries are easier to establish when things are going well.

If you find yourself in a relationship in which there is disrespect or abuse, then the question to ask is "What am I doing that is giving you the impression that I will tolerate or accept these behaviors?" This can begin the dialogue that leads to better understanding and the establishment of clear and healthy boundaries. It is important to recognize that boundaries are for you, not for the other person. If the expectation is that when you state your boundaries, the other person will stop the unacceptable behaviors, this is not a boundary: this is an attempt to control. A boundary is to protect you and to give you options for self-care.

In this story, boundary setting alleviated distress ...

Josie and Penny looked forward to meeting for lunch once per month as a commitment to making the time in their busy schedules to support their friendship. Josie would arrive a few minutes early and then wait impatiently until Penny would run in breathlessly with one excuse or another for her tardiness. Josie began to recognize her feeling of frustration, which would start building hours before, in anticipation of Penny's lateness. Josie realized that if she continued to fume on the inside, Penny would have no idea of the aggravation that Josie was stuffing. Josie realized that she would have to risk the discomfort of establishing a boundary with Penny.

The next time they met for lunch, Josie explained to Penny the distress she had been experiencing from Penny's lack of punctuality. Penny's immediate reaction was to justify her tardiness with the usual excuses of people who are oblivious of the importance of other people's time. Josie curtailed the rebuttal by offering other options. Josie suggested that if

Penny's other responsibilities made it impractical for her to commit to a specific time for lunch, then perhaps they could choose another activity that was more flexible. They were able to come up with creative solutions, such as meeting at a gallery showing, when Josie could begin to view the artwork and there was no longer a sense of waiting for Penny to arrive. Interestingly, as time went by, Penny's on-time record improved dramatically.

Josie learned to apply what she had learned from the situation with Penny to her relationship with her mother. Josie's childhood was marred by many distressing situations caused by her alcoholic father's behaviors. Josie, despite her parents' strong disapproval, made a decision. She went away to a college in another state, rather than to the local college of their choice. Josie distanced herself from the chaos and had no contact with them for five years.

When Josie's father died of complications from his alcoholism, she tried to reestablish contact with her mother. Josie faced another harsh reality. Over time, her mother had succumbed to the same compulsion. Her mother's drinking had increased significantly.

It was not possible to have a lucid phone conversation with her mother after five o'clock in the evening. Josie's attempt to spend a few days with her mother was so disturbing that Josie vowed never to put herself through that experience again. She came up with a compromise to make it possible for her to reconnect with her mother. She set the boundary that she would stay in a hotel nearby. She would go over each morning and spend enjoyable time with her mother, and then she would return to her hotel around three o'clock. She explained honestly to her mother the rationale behind this decision, and the topic was not discussed again.

With the realization that there was nothing else she could do, Josie honored her feelings of sadness and then moved on to accept her mother without change and to love her unconditionally. Once Josie established the boundaries, she could continue to hope and pray that her mother would find the freedom and joy of sobriety.

> We can say what we need to say. We can
> gently, but assertively, speak our mind. We do
> not need to be judgmental, tactless, blaming
> or cruel when we speak our truths.
> —Melody Beattie

The concept of your GPO score can disrupt your boundary setting. It is important to recognize feelings of guilt, pity, or obligation (GPO). The idea for this acronym came from the analogy of a GPA score. You want a high GPA score in school but a low GPO score in your relationships. You give yourself a high GPO score when you recognize that guilt, pity, or obligation drive your behaviors. You feel you *should* or *have to* do something for someone, and you generally feel resentful and unappreciated afterward. You complain that you are always doing things for other people, yet you have no boundaries to guide them. You may get some grim satisfaction from being the person who everyone comes to for help. Boundaries help you recognize when others may try to manipulate you through guilt, pity, or obligation.

Responsible adults strive to meet true obligations, such as parenting, family, work, and social ones. When you think it through, you often discover there are "obligations" you are not obliged to do. You deny your own needs and experience anger later if others do not meet your expectations. There are times when the best way to help is not to help. Free of the need to "fix" everything and everybody, you learn that it is counterproductive to do for others what they can and need to do for themselves.

There are occasions when the answer *no* is muffled and replaced by an impulsive *yes*. Eventually you learn that when you say yes to something you do not want to do, you are saying no to something that is really important to you. You determine the value of each precious moment. When you discover that saying no does not make you a bad person, saying no can be peaceful and loving. You learn that "No" is a complete sentence. You do not have to create an elaborate story to justify your no. The other person does not need to hear that your fictitious aunt Hilda is passing though from Nebraska for one night and you can't miss seeing her. A simple no, perhaps with a suggestion for another convenient time, will suffice. You also accept that the other person may not be happy with your decision.

There are occasions when you choose to help, and you do so from a different perspective, without attachment. You give, simply to give, knowing that this is the right thing to do at that time. There is no residual resentment because you are free of any GPO.

You move toward having clear, consistent, flexible, healthy boundaries in your life today, to foster supportive relationships. You begin by questioning the type of boundaries that existed in your family of origin. Were they too rigid, too unpredictable, too loose, or perhaps there were no boundaries? Too rigid might foster external compliance for a while but will mimic attempts to control and invite distance and defensiveness. Boundaries that are too loose are useless because they are not taken seriously. Boundaries need to be firm enough to provide physical and emotional safety and at the same time flexible enough to nurture love and understanding.

In a parent-child situation, there is the parent who, in a moment of anger, impulsively sets unreasonable boundaries for a minor infraction, such as, "You are grounded for a month—no TV, no friends, no cell phone or games." An hour later when the child asks if he can go next door to see his friend's new game from his father, the parent thoughtlessly says, "Okay." At the other end of the spectrum, there is the parent whose boundary is carved in stone, and a child's pleading to go with the family to his grandmother's seventieth birthday celebration is firmly denied.

There needs to be flexibility and moderation, making allowance for gray areas to avoid extremes. Boundaries are meant to be loving, respectful, and kind. The benefit of having healthy boundaries is that you are responsible to each other but not for each other. Boundaries are designed to provide safety, structure, and security.

> Your life does not get better by chance,
> it gets better by change.
> —Jim Rohn

Key Points

- Breathe.

- Take the time to determine what you want, rather than only what you don't want.

  Begin by validating what is working in the relationship and invite the discussion on what is important in the relationship. Take the time to understand each other's thoughts and feelings, to identify what is helpful and what is not. Discuss if each is committed to working on personal change for self-care and to strengthen the relationship. This takes time and effort. It has been said that a lack of boundaries can foster a lack of respect.

- Be calm and certain that you have thought it through.

Give yourself the time and space to thoroughly think through the boundaries you are about to set. Have the conversation when both are feeling calm and grounded. Make sure that these are reasonable and attainable. Getting feedback from reliable sources can provide input you may not have considered. Be prepared to come from a peaceful place of love rather than reacting impulsively in a moment of anger or pain. Seldom is anything heard or accomplished when the words are fueled by anger.

When you have clarified your intention, discuss and firmly establish together the boundary or boundaries and the consequences if the boundaries are not respected. Be sure that you are able to and will follow through on these consequences, if indeed the boundaries cannot be met. Failure to follow through will destroy credibility. Repetitive threats such as "If you keep doing this, I'm leaving" become meaningless if nothing changes. Consequences have to be well thought out and solution focused.

- Understand that boundaries are designed to achieve clarity; boundaries are not rules.

Boundaries are not futile attempts to control. Boundaries are protection against resentment. You need to know ahead of time how to take care of yourself if the other is incapable or unwilling to join you in a place of mutual respect. You also allow room for flexibility as events unfold.

- Be prepared for any response, without taking responsibility or judging.

Boundaries are for you, and you have no guarantee of how the other person will react. When you are clear that you want to have healthy boundaries in all your relationships, you will create a healthy, like-minded social support system. Some people are able to stay the course, while others may choose to walk away. If the latter happens, you learn from the experience and move on.

- Be patient with yourself and others as the process of change unfolds.

Life is constantly giving you opportunities to learn and grow as you go through this process of change. This requires awareness, openness, humility, and acceptance, which is enhanced by honest communication and validation of positive changes. It may take time and patience to explore situations that can unexpectedly take you back to old behaviors. Each time, you will have an opportunity to increase your understanding and strengthen your commitment to change. You expect the same behaviors from yourself that you are asking from others. You observe other healthy relationships and invite feedback on what is working for them. You are worth it, the others in your life are worth it, and life becomes more rewarding.

Boundaries include the three Rs:

- respect for self
- respect for others
- responsibility for all your actions

Examine your relationship to determine what you can and cannot tolerate and establish the healthy boundaries that you will follow through on. Explore these boundaries together and discuss what is acceptable to both parties. Remember that boundaries are not rules, and there is no guarantee that they will be respected. Know how you will protect yourself if these boundaries cannot be met.

One idea is to look at boundaries the way you plan for hurricanes; you know what to do if a hurricane hits, and you do not waste time worrying in advance. Boundaries are established when you are in a calm, peaceful place.

Healthy relationships require healthy boundaries that will be revisited and adjusted from time to time.

CHAPTER 18

Discover the Freedom of Forgiveness

> Forgive others, not because they deserve
> forgiveness, but because you deserve peace.
> —Jonathan Lockwood Hule

Forgiveness is a highly emotional topic. Forgiving has been described in the 1976 book *A Course in Miracles* as the pathway to happiness and the quickest way to undo suffering and pain. As such, choosing not to forgive is a decision to suffer. Forgive and let it go.

Forgiveness is one of the most difficult concepts to grasp. Some actions might seem unforgivable until you realize that forgiveness does not make it right, nor does forgiveness absolve anyone of wrongdoing. Forgiveness frees you from attachment to the hurt you experienced. If you have dragged this pain along for a long time, it may seem like such an integral part of your being that you cannot imagine being free of this albatross on your back.

The willingness to discover the freedom of forgiveness opens the door to inner peace. This cannot be accomplished by repressing old pain and striving to bury the past or by fanning the flames of your suffering. Leave the hurtful behavior in the past where it belongs, so that it does not continue to torment you today. Do not delay forgiving until the offenders apologize, or because they are no longer present in your life or they don't care. Accept that forgiveness will bring the healing your heart yearns for.

> Forgiveness doesn't excuse their actions. Forgiveness
> stops their actions from destroying your heart.
> —Karen Salmansohn

Lewis Smedes's well-known book *Forgive and Forget* provides an excellent road map through the stages of forgiveness. "My hurt brings me into the first stage of forgiving—the critical stage at which I had to make a simple decision: Did I want to be healed or did I want to go on suffering from an unfair hurt lodged in my memory?"

Smedes makes a distinction among types of hurt; there are the minor annoyances and disappointments that we can easily let go, but there is deeper pain caused by disloyalty, betrayal, and brutality.

The most powerful thing I can change is my perception.

Your perception of the event or events is an important factor. Great care must be taken with the words you use to record the event. Consider the hurt caused by disloyalty versus the more devastating word, betrayal. In the Bible story (Luke 22) of Jesus and his disciples, Peter was disloyal to Jesus when he denied knowing him. Judas betrayed him when he delivered him to his enemies. Certainly, betrayal would be more intensely hurtful. If everything is labeled "horrible" and "awful," then there will be many more things to forgive.

When you reflect on the situation and rethink your immediate thoughts and feelings, there will be times when forgiveness is easier or may not even be necessary.

When there is deep pain, sometimes you just don't know what to do, and these are options. You can wish there was a way to go back in time and erase the painful event (which isn't possible), keep reinforcing the justified anger and maintain the toxic resentment (creating disease), or go through the emotional work to touch your thoughts and feelings with compassion, revisit and resolve the painful memory to empower you to forgive (challenging, worthwhile, and sometimes painful).

The emotional work can be compared to having an old wound that continues to fester and making the decision to reopen the wound, clear out the infection, and apply the medication to promote healing. In this analogy, the decision would be to reopen the unresolved emotional pain, do the therapeutic work to explore and clear out the suffering, and apply the medication of forgiveness to promote healing and freedom.

> Our deepest wounds, when integrated,
> become our greatest strength.
> —Mariette Hartley

From Lewis Smedes's book *Forgive and Forget* comes "The Magic Eyes—A Little Fable":

> In the village of Faken in innermost Friesland there lived a long thin baker named Fouke, a righteous man, with a long thin chin and a long thin nose. Fouke was so upright that he seemed to spray righteousness from his thin lips over everyone who came near him; so the people of Faken preferred to stay away.
>
> Fouke's wife, Hilda, was short and round, her arms were round, her bosom was round, and her rump was round. Hilda did not keep people at bay with righteousness; her soft

roundness seemed to invite them instead to come close to her in order to share the warm cheer of her open heart.

Hilda respected her righteous husband, and loved him too, as much as he allowed her; but her heart ached for something more from him than his worthy righteousness. And there, in the bed of her need, lay the seed of sadness. One morning, having worked since dawn to knead his dough for the ovens, Fouke came home and found a stranger in his bedroom lying on Hilda's round bosom. Hilda's adultery soon became the talk of the tavern and the scandal of the Faken congregation. Everyone assumed that Fouke would cast Hilda out of his house, so righteous was he. But he surprised everyone by keeping Hilda as his wife, saying he forgave her as the Good Book said he should.

In his heart of hearts, however, Fouke could not forgive Hilda for bringing shame to his name. Whenever he thought about her, his feelings toward her were angry and hard; he despised her as if she were a common whore. When it came right down to it, he hated her for betraying him after he had been so good and so faithful a husband to her. He only pretended to forgive Hilda so that he could punish her with his righteous mercy.

But Fouke's fakery did not sit well in heaven. So each time that Fouke would feel his secret hatred toward Hilda, an angel came to him and dropped a small pebble, hardly the size of a shirt button, into Fouke's heart. Each time a pebble dropped, Fouke would feel a stab of pain like the pain he felt the moment he came on Hilda feeding her hungry heart from a stranger's larder. Thus he hated her the more; his hate brought him pain and his pain made him hate.

The pebbles multiplied. And Fouke's heart grew very heavy with the weight of them, so heavy that the top half of his body bent forward so far that he had to strain his neck upward in order to see straight ahead.

Weary with hurt, Fouke began to wish he were dead. The angel who dropped the pebbles into his heart came to Fouke one night and told him how he could be healed of his hurt. There was one remedy, he said, only one, for the hurt of a wounded heart. Fouke would need the miracle of the magic eyes.

The fable concludes with Fouke's transformation. Fouke had carried this hatred so long knowing that nothing could change the past; it took a while until his heavy pain compelled him to ask the angel for the magic eyes. The angel granted Fouke's request and advised him that he could heal the hurt from the past only with the visual perception of the magic eyes. Each time he saw Hilda through new eyes, a pebble would be lifted until his heart grew lighter. With this freedom, Fouke was unburdened and he invited his loving, fallible wife, Hilda, into his heart again.

As you reflect on the fable, you can empathize with Fouke's deep pain. Yet it was sad to see how his justified anger grew into hatred and vengeance toward Hilda for betraying him. This completely blocked the path to the healing and restoration of their marriage. Only when he was guided to self-compassion and the compassion to see a simple, kindhearted woman who had done something wrong, could they be free of the old pain and open to all possibilities. Are there "unforgivable" events in your past that could also be healed through the power of forgiveness and free you from suffering?

To err is human, to forgive divine.
—Alexander Pope

There is a well-known story that illustrates the power of forgiveness, about a young Jewish man, Joey Riklis, from Cleveland, Ohio, who goes to visit the Wailing Wall in Jerusalem after his father had died.

His father had been a survivor of the holocaust and was an ardent practitioner of his Jewish faith. Joey had rebelled against his father's faith, and the two of them had been alienated for some time. He was feeling guilt and remorse over his father's death and blamed himself for it. Joey had traveled to India and done his share of guru hopping in hopes of finding an alternative to his Hebrew religious heritage. But nothing truly satisfied or filled his spiritual longing. So he went to Israel to explore the heritage that he had formerly spurned. While there, he noticed people scribbling notes on small pieces of paper and inserting them into the crevices of the Wailing Wall.

He asked a young man there what this was about and was told that they were petitionary prayers. People believed the stones were so holy that any requests placed inside of them would be especially blessed.

So Joey decided to write his own petition, addressed to his father. He wrote, "Dear Father, I beg you to forgive me for the pain I caused you. I loved you very much and I will never forget you. And please know that nothing that you taught me was in vain. I will not betray your family's deaths. I promise."

Joey searched for an empty crevice in the wall to place his petition. There were notes crammed and overflowing everywhere in the wall. After an hour of trying to find an empty space, he finally found a spot and inserted his small note into the crack. As he did so, he accidentally dislodged another that had been resting there, and it fell to the ground. He bent down and picked it up and was going to put it back when he was overcome by a strong impulse to open the note and read it, which he did. Here is what he read: "My Dear Son Joey, If you should ever happen to come to Israel and somehow miraculously find this note, this is what I want you to know: I always loved you even when you hurt me, and I will never stop loving you. You are, and always will be, my beloved son. And Joey, please know that I forgive you for everything, and only hope that you in turn will forgive a foolish old man." Signed, Adam Riklis, Cleveland, Ohio.

Joey's father's freedom began several years before Joey's, from the moment he forgave Joey and then went on to seek forgiveness for himself. If you hold on to the belief that you cannot forgive the ones who hurt you until they admit they were wrong and apologize, you give them the power to keep you trapped in old pain. Forgiveness opens the trapdoor and sets you free.

When you understand that prolonged anger with someone hurts only you, you learn how to let go of your anger—not for the other person but for yourself. This does not mean that once you forgive, you also forget. Forgiving makes it possible for you to accept that it happened, that you can't go back and change what happened; it is over, and you can let go. One of the most loved and often-spoken prayers is the Lord's Prayer, which equates seeking forgiveness with forgiving others: "Forgive us our trespasses as we forgive those who trespass against us." Thus you forgive as you would like to be forgiven.

Forgiveness is man's deepest need and greatest achievement.
—Horace Bushnell

Forgiveness of self and others is a process. Self-forgiveness brings you out of the shadows and lights the path to being wiser today than you were in the past. This can be your restart button to get unstuck and move on. Guidelines in chapter 20, "Transform Regrets and Remorse," can help you follow through on your decision to forgive yourself.

In his talk to more than ten thousand listeners in Australia in 2013, the Dalai Lama invited all to practice forgiveness, simply a way of respecting your own physical health enough to not allow negative feelings to cause you harm. You learn to forgive by practicing forgiveness.

There was a subtle message for our young viewers in Walt Disney's remake of *Cinderella*; as Cinderella was leaving with the prince, she looked back at her wicked stepmother and said, "I forgive you." Thus she was able to move forward to her new chapter, unencumbered by bitterness and anger, and she could realign with her mother's wise counsel, "Have courage and be kind." Going through the stages of forgiveness can lead to freedom, when all is forgiven and all is love.

Key Points

- Breathe.
- Reflect on the people or situations you have been unable to forgive.
- Identify and change the thinking that keeps you trapped in hatred and blocks your willingness to forgive.
- Replace this faulty thinking with the understanding that forgiveness heals your heart and soul.

- Do the emotional work to free your heart of the undeserved pain, and forgive for your own peace and happiness.
- Remember that forgiveness includes self-forgiveness.

You have a lot less to forgive when you don't take things personally.

You can begin your process by exploring whether the pain you are experiencing now is coming from what happened, or is this pain coming from holding on to what happened. It's been said that the most difficult anger to let go of is justified anger. Understanding is the path to forgiveness, and forgiveness is the path to healing. Thus you free yourself of the pain you never deserved through the healing power of forgiveness. You can choose to restore the relationship or walk away peacefully and reopen your beautiful heart to receive life's blessings.

CHAPTER 19

Review, Resolve, and Release Resentments

When you harbor bitterness, happiness will dock elsewhere.
—Andy Rooney

Resent comes from the French *resentir*, to feel all over again, and the Latin *sentir*, to perceive. Resentment can continue to harm you long after the hurtful event occurred. It takes mental and emotional energy to maintain the hostility by reliving the painful past over and over.

Burying the resentment is also harmful, as you dismiss your pain and build a wall that shuts everything out. Holding on to the justified anger, or burying it, gets in the way of resolving and releasing suffering and blocks the flow of life. Either way, you are giving greater power to those who wronged you as you drag all the pain, strain, and negativity from one moment to the next.

Your tormentor today is yourself left over from yesterday.
—Deepak Chopra

This is a story of holding on to resentment. Two war veterans, Sam and Vince, ran into each other for the first time since their imprisonment in the same POW camp. They revisited their horrific experiences and reflected on how war can bring out the worst and best in people. As they were parting, Sam asked the question, "After all these years, how do you feel about those prison guards?"

Vince's response was quick and harsh. "I will always hate them for their cruelty and everything they did to us."

Sam was struck by the intense rage and fury he heard and said quietly, "Then I guess you will always be their prisoner." Vince had never found the way to let go of his justified anger and desire for revenge. He was unaware of the amount of energy it took to carry this resentment and the toll this toxicity was taking on his physical, emotional, and spiritual well-being. He had kept suffering alive long after his release and wore his badge of victimhood every day.

When a heart attack almost ended his life, Vince's wife and children begged him to get help to deal with his resentments. Through therapy, Vince learned that he would never have a whole, fulfilling life until he resolved his unfinished business. He gained the understanding that getting revenge never gets revenge. As he freed his heart of resentments, he made room for the love of his family.

> Resentment is like taking poison and
> waiting for the other person to die.
> —Adapted by AA from Emmet Fox, *Sermon on the Mount*

Compare this to another story told by Dalai Lama. I had the privilege of seeing him when he was the guest speaker at a conference at Florida International University in Miami. The Dalai Lama spoke of a Tibetan monk he met who had been in a Chinese gulag or prison, where he was brutally tortured, placed in solitary confinement, and prohibited from practicing his traditions for more than twenty years. The Dalai Lama asked him what his greatest fear had been during all those years. One would think the response would have been fear of death or fear of increased torture. The monk replied that his fear was that he would lose compassion for his Chinese jailers! For this monk, the greatest loss would be the loss of compassion for all living creatures.

What is remarkable is that the monk did not continue to suffer after his release; he emerged intact, peaceful, and ready to continue his work of giving back to the world. His freedom from imprisonment was accompanied by freedom from resentment.

> As I walked out the door toward the gate that
> would lead to my freedom, I knew that if I didn't
> leave my bitterness behind, I'd still be in prison.
> —Nelson Mandela

Everyone has a personal story of pain that was never deserved and the choice to hold on to the resentment or learn how to let go and grow. Janice had had her own share of struggles with alcohol. One evening, during a sober period in her life, she began a conversation with a young man who suggested that they continue their discussion over a beer. Several hours later, Janice was awakened by horrified neighbors, who had discovered her because her little dog had been running around and barking frantically to get someone to come to her apartment. Her friends' phone numbers were found in her cell phone, and they rushed over and called 911. They took photographs of her badly beaten body with her cell phone. The day she showed me the photos of her battered body, it was difficult for me to even look at them.

Janice was filled with rage as she thought about the brutal attack that could have ended her life except for the bravery of her little dog. She felt great sadness that her dog had been traumatized by watching her being raped and brutally beaten. Other old, unresolved resentments began to surface.

She remembered the hurtful things her father had said to her when she disclosed her sexual orientation, his rejection and her despair when her mother had been unable to defend her. She realized that she needed professional help, and she began the process.

Her parents supported her financially for treatment, and in time her father participated to address his own unresolved anger issues. At one point in treatment, Janice had been furious at being blamed because of a misunderstanding. As we were speaking, I went to gently touch her shoulder. She recoiled and asked me not to touch her when she was angry. I validated her for her awareness and ability to set this boundary. It helped me recognize the smoldering rage that lurked right below the surface.

Janice threw herself into her treatment process and began the painful journey of revisiting old pain, and step-by-step letting go of anger and shame. The dreaded day of the trial, she hardly recognized her attacker. It seemed like a vague, surreal experience, because of her physical and emotional state at that time. She continued the crucial work and a year later made the decision to visit her attacker in prison to take responsibility for her part and to let go of her resentment toward him. She apologized for being the person who drank with him and allowed him into her home, which then unleashed his addiction monster and escalated to the vicious attack that took place in a blackout.

She was surprised how young her attacker was and vaguely remembered seeing him in her neighborhood. The young man broke down into tears and promised her that his time in prison would be used to make amends and change his life so that never again would he hurt anyone. This experience strengthened her commitment to do whatever it took to release resentments, transcend suffering, and heal.

She incorporated the Buddhist philosophy "The mind is our obstacle, not the past."

After working through the physical and psychological distress, Janice came to terms with the traumatic event as the starting point of the path from PTSD (post-traumatic stress disorder) to PTG (post-traumatic growth). She would not only bounce back, she would bounce forward. Her capacity to bring meaning to this horrific experience allowed her to explore new opportunities.

Another year later, Janice went back to school and completed her degree in counseling. She transformed her painful experience into the reason for helping others, and she was empowered to evolve into a compassionate healer. Janice's father did something totally unexpected. He continued his own therapy, discarded all the excuses, and expressed his sorrow for the way he had treated her. When love replaces fear, the healing begins.

> I am more vulnerable than I thought, but
> much stronger that I ever imagined.
> —Tedeschi and Calhoun

These famous words from Viktor Frankl continue to inspire us:

> We who lived in the concentration camps can remember the men who walked through the huts comforting others, giving away their last piece of bread. They may have been few in number, but they offer sufficient proof that everything can be taken from a man but one thing: the last of the human freedoms— to choose one's attitude in any given set of circumstances, to choose one's own way. A

thought transfixed me: for the first time in my life I saw the truth as it is set into song by so many poets, proclaimed as the final wisdom by so many thinkers. The truth—that love is the ultimate and the highest goal to which man can aspire.

I do not forget any good deed done to me &
I do not carry a grudge for a bad one.
—Viktor E. Frankl, *Man's Search for Meaning*

This is a story about deep, unprocessed resentment and the impact of an unexpected trigger. Richard grew up with an alcoholic father whose behaviors went through three stages when he was drinking. The first stage was the silly and vulgar humor that was offensive to his wife and sons. The second stage, he became hostile and aggressive, and the third stage he passed out, and his family felt the temporary relief from the cessation of the abusive behaviors.

Richard shared about one occasion when his father was in the second, rageful stage. When Richard shouted at him to stop verbally abusing his mother, his father lunged toward him, shoved him forcefully in the chest, and proceeded to punch him unmercifully. Richard's body healed, but he buried his emotional pain for ten years and never spoke of the hatred he felt for his father.

One afternoon, Richard was having a friendly debate with his best friend, Charlie, about their favorite sports teams. Charlie gave Richard a playful shove, commenting that Richard's sports team were losers. Charlie was shocked when Richard broke down sobbing and collapsed on the floor. The similarity of a shove triggered Richard's subconscious, and past and present merged. A dark curtain had been lifted, and Richard felt the overwhelming anguish from his father's violent behaviors during his childhood. It was as if years of frozen anger had thawed and erupted into a landslide. When he calmed himself, Richard haltingly explained what had happened to a bewildered Charlie. Having exposed his pent-up emotions, Richard knew he could no longer contain his seething hatred; he had to seek help.

Fear will often block any attempts to revisit the past until you realize that the event did not kill you and facing the shadow won't kill you either. By exploring and resolving his painful childhood, Richard released the resentments and later reconnected with his aging father, who was terminally ill and remorseful. Richard felt as if a heavy block had been lifted from his heart and replaced with light and love.

> And the day came when the risk to remain tight in a bud
> was more painful than the risk it took to blossom.
> —Anais Nin

A speaker compared carrying resentments to walking through a crowded airport burdened with heavy luggage. Today you can decide to take all the steps to travel light by reviewing and releasing the past, to get out of the exhausting cycle of hatred, guilt, and victimhood. Make peace with the past so that you can flourish in the present.

Nell's story shows the need to stop recharging old anger. Nell would retell endless stories of all the hurtful things her husband had done. Nell recounted the day her sister finally stopped her and asked, "Can you see that constant whining takes you from being a victim to being a volunteer for the miserable life you say you are living? Imagine how your life could change and what you could learn if you would resolve the past and take responsibility for your part of the problem and the solution." Nell listened quietly, knowing that her sister was trying to help her. She learned how to shift her attention to unload the heaviness of her resentments and lighten her path.

You can also apply this process to healing your soul and the world. Learn from older people whose experiences made them wise or made them bitter. Replace the lament "Why me, God? Why is this happening to me?" with Cathy's prayer, "God, please help me learn the lesson well and quickly so that I can grow and move on."

> Do you think peace of mind can be found in holding
> a grudge ... or harboring resentment ... or wallowing
> in thoughts of what could have been? Me neither.
> —Dr. Steven Maraboli

Key Points

- Breathe.
- Be willing to release resentments.
- Identify the root cause. List the people and events.
- Honor your feelings.
- Find your path to healing—therapy, support groups, prayer, introspection.
- Learn to let go of resentment for the past, anger in the present, and fear for the future.
- Visualize a life free of resentments.
- Accept your vulnerability and your resilience.
- Recognize the cyclical nature of healing and the possibility of resolving an old issue again at a deeper level.
- Validate your commitment to peace.

Per ardua ad astra—through adversity to the stars. This became the motto of the Royal Air Force and other

Commonwealth air forces in 1912. This would be an excellent mantra to help you observe, process, accept, and let go, to be able to live a life free of resentments. Rather than constantly replaying the negative memories, change the channel to pleasant memories. Celebrate your victory of moving through hate and pain to light and love.

CHAPTER 20

Transform Regret and Remorse

The beauty of life is, while we cannot undo what is done,
we can see it, understand it, learn from it and change.
So that every new moment is spent, not in regret, guilt,
fear or anger, but in wisdom, understanding and love.
—Jennifer Edwards

Everyone can look back with regret about having done something in the past or not having done something that should or could have been done. In relationships, the deeper the love and affection, the more intense the feelings of regret may become.

Regret comes from the French *regreter*, to lament. You look at the consequences and wish you had the chance to go back and do something differently. This can occur, for example, when you look back at your child's irresponsible behaviors that could have been corrected with more discipline or boundaries, and now the child has passed the stage of parental influence.

There can also be hurtful words that you wish had never escaped your lips, because of the pain that resulted. Regret keeps you trapped in the past, especially when compounded by grief after a major loss, and there is nothing you can do to fix it or change it now.

This story shows that it is vital to have self-compassion,

patience, and acceptance. Charlene struggled with regret after the loss of her sister, Sandra. They enjoyed a wonderful sibling relationship, and when Sandra was diagnosed with a terminal illness, they focused on a cure. As Sandra's illness progressed, they continued to live in the possibility of her recovery. When Sandra passed away peacefully one afternoon, Charlene received the phone call with sorrow and disbelief. She had lost her only sister, loving friend, and last sibling.

Looking back, she wished they had recognized what limited time Sandra had and that they had spent more time embracing the present moment.

Charlene found herself ruminating on all the things they could have done together, despite Sandra's limitations. When regrets became too consuming, Charlene realized that she would have to shift her focus to the many things they had enjoyed, like the mornings that they sat beside the canal and enjoyed nature or the board games they had played. Eventually, Charlene also let go of her frustration with all the doctors, tests, and hospital visits that could not cure her sister's disease.

During a conversation with her sister's son, Stan, Charlene drifted into the past. Stan had just shared about his commitment to stay in the light and his growing awareness of how his life was changing as a result of this shift in consciousness. As he listened to Charlene bring up her sadness from the missed opportunities with her sister, he cautioned her that regret keeps you away from the light and that to walk in the light you must let go of regret. She thanked him for the reminder and returned to gratitude for their journey together.

Every experience is a learning opportunity. Charlene decided that she would use past regrets to guide action in the present. Keeping in mind that hindsight is twenty-twenty, she would look at each situation from the perspective of five years in the future. Looking back, what would she wish she had done differently?

A year later, Charlene was given an opportunity. Her sister's son, Jon, was diagnosed with stage four lung cancer, complicated with emphysema and other health issues. She determined that five years from now, she would regret not having made the time to go to visit him. Charlene invited her son and his partner to travel with her, and they made arrangements to spend a weekend together. It was a very rewarding experience with quality time. In fact, Charlene got another occasion to spend time with Jon along with his brother, Stan. Her last phone conversation with Jon took place thirty minutes before his death. She was deeply grateful for their time together. She also felt that comforting her sister's son was a way to honor her sister.

Happiness is the art of never holding in your mind the memory of any unpleasant things that have happened.
—Gautama Buddha

Remorse, which often accompanies regret, is taking responsibility and being accountable for your actions, with a sincere desire to change and to do things differently. There is sadness and genuine sorrow for the pain you caused. The origin of remorse is the Anglo French *mordant*, biting. Something comes back to bite you, and you experience guilt and anguish.

Anita had to resolve feelings of remorse. After many years of living with a husband who struggled with addiction, she became increasingly frustrated and discouraged. A wonderful man when he was sober, this was overshadowed by the many times when he was impaired. She lost the ability to enjoy his positive actions, which were overshadowed by the underlying dread of the next relapse. She loved him for the wonderful person she knew he was, yet the constant disappointments ate away the fabric of her happiness.

One morning, Anita's husband did not wake up. She felt as if this was a bad dream as she watched the Fire Rescue team take over. When they were unable to revive her husband, waves of disbelief, despair, anger, remorse, and sorrow threatened to overwhelm her. She heard the voice in her head chastising her for each harsh remark she had made and for each time that frustration and discouragement had pushed them apart. She kept wondering what more she could have done to save him. She felt the love he had so freely given her, and she let go of the disappointments from his unstable recovery, but she was frozen in her self-blame and self-condemnation.

With time and great effort, Anita accepted that continuing to berate herself would not bring back their time together or give her another chance to appreciate his sober periods. She had forgiven him for the relapses, and she had to forgive herself for her reactions.

Anita also realized that she was delaying the grieving process with this distressing distraction. Her husband was free now and no longer burdened by the addiction he had not been able to overcome. She reached out for the help and support she needed. She took responsibility for all her actions, identified changes she needed to make, and began the process of living a new chapter in her life. She transformed her remorse into helping others in her support group, by sharing what she had learned and wished she had understood sooner.

Suffering is necessary, until you realize it is unnecessary.
—Eckhart Tolle

Whatever happened in the past does not exist today. There are steps to work through and resolve past pain to move freely into the present moment. When you have done all that you can to make amends and change, you accept that it is time to move forward. Each time thoughts of the painful past attempt to mislead you into going back to regret and remorse, you remind yourself, "It doesn't exist"; there is nothing more you can do. Let go and be free.

Often, caring people get stuck in guilt and shame, unable to reconcile the past. The difference between guilt and shame has been explained this way: guilt is feeling that you did something bad; shame is feeling that you are bad. The action or behavior cannot be undone; it is what happens afterward that matters.

When you make the commitment to work through past unresolved issues, you can use the lessons to empower you to make your actions become your living amends.

Holding on to remorse benefits no one and simply contaminates the present. You cannot change what happened in the past, and each new day brings opportunities to practice new behaviors. Validate each change and recognize how new behaviors bring new outcomes.

A man should never be ashamed to own that he has been in the wrong, which is but saying in other words that he is wiser today than he was yesterday.
—Alexander Pope

You can only share what you have inside. If you clog up your soul with negativity and self-blame, then you will have only negativity and blame to give to others. Those who cling to the shameful behavior from the past often become shameless in the way they treat others, and the devastating pattern goes from generation to generation.

If you want to see the daylight, you have to open the drapes. Take responsibility for your actions; you have to claim them to change them. Explore all the aspects of your poor choices to identify the lesson and grow from mistakes. When you learn from every experience, yours or someone else's, you can apply that learning whenever similar situations arise, even those that may be packaged differently.

Watch your thoughts. You have no control over the first thought that comes up uninvited. You can breathe and observe the thought to determine if it moves you toward your goals or drags you back to the troubled past. You have the choice to reinforce the thought or gently and firmly let it go. The longer you hold the thought, the more ingrained and consuming it becomes.

Be careful when guilt or shame propels you to confess your wrongdoing and apologize to the offended party. This can lead to healing or to unexpected, deep hurt. When all parties are aware of the transgressions, the expression of sorrow, along with the promise and evidence of changed behavior, can lead to reconciliation and restoration of trust. On the other hand, if disclosing this information would only relieve your heavy burden by dumping this on the unsuspecting person and cause unnecessary pain, then take another path. Use these negative emotions to motivate personal transformation. You will stop feeling guilty or ashamed when you stop doing the things that made you feel guilty or ashamed. Your actions reveal the sincerity and power of your intention.

There is another method to release persistent, frozen emotions, which are usually about irreversible past events. The preparation step is to explore the event or events from all perspectives to achieve resolution and the willingness to let go of suffering. In this process, you make the time and space to be still and allow your inner self to intentionally and gently witness the surge of pent-up emotions as they intensify, staying with them until they subside and finally diminish. The mind will try to seduce you into stopping, rationalizing that you've done enough for now and can come back to it later. Let go of all thinking (the mind) and keep gently bringing yourself back to what is going on inside you (the body) as feelings lessen and eventually drift away into the emptiness, making room for positive emotions.

This concept is not to be confused with ruminating, where the mind keeps you stuck in the drama. Instead this is the process of allowing rather than resisting the feelings, and the conscious acceptance ultimately dispels the feelings. These feelings often come along with a physical symptom, like heaviness in the chest area for example. As the symptom lightens, this will be a good indication that the feelings are lessening.

It can be helpful to do this exercise with another caring person. It is not necessary to disclose the events that brought the feelings. Discussing the events, which involves the mind, would not be a part of this exercise and would be done at another time, should you choose to do so. The simple gift of each other's quiet presence can enhance this special time of sitting patiently with feelings, which may ebb and flow until they float away. This process can also be guided by a therapist, who can gently encourage you along the way to stay with the feelings until they dissipate.

It is heartening that when you observe the feelings later, everything seems so much lighter. It can be like driving mindfully through a heavy rainstorm and eventually moving on to the clear skies, leaving the downpour behind.

If you have behaved badly, repent, make what amends you can and address yourself to the task of behaving better next time. On no account brood over your wrongdoing. Rolling in the muck is not the best way of getting clean.
—Aldous Huxley, *Brave New World*

Key Points

- Breathe.
- Face and process what you did, or failed to do, and let go of blame and shame.
- Take responsibility for your actions.
- Sincerely apologize when this is beneficial for all concerned.
- Make the time and space for the process of sitting patiently with your feelings until they lessen and drift away.
- Validate each step that you take to release regret and remorse.
- Transform guilt into action for positive change.

Recognize when remorse and regret become the walls of your own prison. Only you can take down these walls, with positive change, acceptance, and self-compassion. Learn from the past and flourish in the present as you endeavor to create the person you want to become. Knowing that perfection is not attainable, strive to be the best you—and be gentle with yourself.

CHAPTER 21

Truth—The Oldest Virtue

To thine own self be true.
—William Shakespeare

Your right hand is raised, and your left hand rests on the Bible. You are asked, "Do you swear to tell the truth, the whole truth, and nothing but the truth, so help you God?" Definition of the simple truth? What you say is true corresponds to the way things actually are. Can this be a way of life?

Many people seem to see truth as influenced by perception or opinion. In response to the opening quote on truth, several people expressed the thinking that truth was a matter of perspective and that truth was different for different people. What is the relationship among truth, reality, and fact, and is it possible to keep these free of judgment, belief, and adaptation?

Definition of the simple lie? What you say is true does not correspond to the way things actually are. Each lie can create stress and anxiety. When lying becomes a pattern, you lose creditability with family and friends and yourself, even at times when you are telling the truth. This negatively impacts your self-esteem, and you feel rejected. There are many justifications for telling lies, even though in most cases lies only delay the exposure of the truth. When the lie is eventually revealed, the hurt from whatever was being hidden is exacerbated by the lies, and fragile trust is once again damaged. The damaging effects show up in the disclosure by a young man named Jack, who said, "I lie to everyone, even to myself."

This story is an example of how quickly lies can take over. Henry recalled a situation when he decided to reconnect with his toxic, former wife. As he was driving to meet her for the first time since their divorce, he received a call from his sister. Fearing that his sister would chastise him for his poor decision, he told her he was on his way to meet a friend. She asked whom, since they had several mutual friends. He responded with the name "Josh." She asked where they were going to meet, and Henry replied that they were meeting for lunch. He felt his chest beginning to tighten. She asked him where they were going to have lunch, and he blurted out the name of a restaurant near where his ex-wife lived. There was a pause, and his sister replied that that particular restaurant had been closed for six months. She told him she had to go and ended the call.

Henry reflected on how easily each lie had led to another lie. In another situation, he would have seen his sister's questions as curiosity, but because he was lying, it felt like interrogation. He realized how quickly he had become swept up in the story he was inventing with each response.

When he later disclosed the truth to his sister, she expressed her frustration and confusion about his need to lie to her and how difficult he made it for her to trust anything he said. Henry wondered if he would ever be able to break his habit of dishonesty. He vowed that he would find his way to truth and honesty. He placed this quote on his mirror to see it every day, so that it would sink into his subconscious and strengthen his resolve: "I am honest and trustworthy."

Gaining trust is like filling a bucket one drop at a time.
—Todd Duncan

One lie can empty that bucket in an instant, and regaining trust will take more time, effort, and commitment.

There was a similar story with Jenny. Jenny wanted to regain her parents' trust and made the decision to strive to be honest and transparent. She would enjoy their conversations during each period of rebuilding trust, until something would occur that would trigger her lies. Her lies would inevitably torpedo the trust she had built and place everything she said under scrutiny again. She would then express her anguish that they didn't trust her.

When she finally stopped blaming her parents for their distrust, she could look inward. She was guided to get in touch with the underlying anxiety that went all the way back to her childhood. She saw how she would automatically revert to manipulating the truth when she was fearful of their disapproval or disappointment. Her shame, unworthiness, and fear of rejection fueled the dishonesty.

Jenny had to face the fact that she would never build an intimate relationship with anyone until she could break through her chronic pattern of dishonesty. She became tired of having everyone she cared about be suspicious of whatever she said, and often not even bother to seek verification. To build her self-esteem, she would have to learn how to tell the truth consistently.

As she approached each new situation, she would have to learn how to take the time to recall exactly what had happened and how this impacted her self-image. This would reinforce her conscious intention of staying aligned with the facts. Doing the "next right thing" took on a deeper meaning, and the process was slow and challenging, as it usually is when striving to break old patterns. Her hope was that one day honesty would be a way of life for her, her new default mode, when she would trust herself and be deserving of trust.

She enlisted the support of others who were on a similar path to consistent truthfulness.

> Oh, what a tangled web we weave ...
> when first we practice to deceive.
> —Walter Scott, *Marmion*

There are many reasons people lie, exaggerate, or manipulate the truth. Common reasons are to look better, to gain respect, to avoid embarrassment, judgment, or consequences, or to escape the discomfort of disclosing unacceptable behaviors. There may be underlying feelings of fear, shame, and guilt, along with the often imperceptible thrill of liar's delight. There is the added tension of having to control facial expression, speech, and body language. This all comes with the high cost of being anxious and guarded most of the time.

Through research, we learn that the brain has to work twice as hard when you are lying. You have to suppress the truth and then fabricate the lie. Research also indicates that the brain consumes 20 percent of the body's total energy. Surely honesty is a far better use of your energy. When you take the time to stop and write your own questions and answers, you gain insight into your triggers.

Beth shared one evening, "I learned that I lie to preserve the social mask I wear, because if I take it off, others will see that I am not perfect, and they may reject me when they find out who I really am."

> Every time we tell a lie, the thing
> that we fear grows stronger.
> —Tad Williams

Throughout nature, there is evidence of deception being

used for survival. Yet, when deception is so ingrained that it becomes a pattern for no apparent reason, this is a barrier to human connection and growth. You tell the first lie you think is necessary, and then there are more lies. You often feel insecure and threatened when someone confronts you because of the inconsistency in your stories. For example, one day you share that you were pulled over for a traffic violation in the morning on the way to work, yet the ticket you got indicated it was at eight o'clock in the evening and marijuana was found in your car.

You know you are ready to break the cycle of deception when you are exhausted with hiding and pretending. With determination, you learn how to slow down and endure the immediate discomfort and overcome the impulse to lie. You recognize the value of honesty, make the commitment to a life of integrity, and become deliberate and thoughtful of everything you say, do, and think.

Today, truth may have become an even more rare and valuable commodity. Once honored and trusted sources, such as officials in high positions, journalists, and reporters on television and newspapers, are now being viewed with great skepticism, and everything reported has to be scrutinized and challenged. This elevates the importance of personal honesty to an even higher level, as an essential part of social interactions, especially intimate, loving relationships. An added incentive for responsible behaviors and truthfulness is the realization that in this age of rapidly advancing technology, privacy has been replaced with publicity. Consider that your personal and professional life is no longer hidden. Just check social media.

If you tell the truth, you don't have to remember anything.
—Mark Twain

Seeking outside help can increase the depth of your understanding and acceptance, stimulate motivation, and provide guidance. Then it will be up to you to stop doing the kinds of things that you would have to lie about later. You cannot do anything to undo past transgressions. You can learn the lessons and strengthen your resolve to embrace truth. You no longer see yourself as a liar, but as someone who has behaved dishonestly in the past, and can change. Let the truth remake your life. Today is the day. Begin now. Speak with the intention of love and truth. Earn the freedom of a life of honesty and self-worth as you build a new track record of reliability over time.

> Being truthful is the new Beautiful.
> —Suzy Kassem

Key Points

- Breathe.
- Slow down and think before your speak.
- Recollect the facts logically.
- Speak with the intention of truth and love.
- Validate your honesty.
- Work on changing unacceptable behaviors.
- Enjoy your freedom.

Your decision to break the negative pattern and strive for a life of honesty will motivate you to identify your strengths and your challenges and apply your energy to becoming the kind of person you want to be.

Rather than hide or ignore what you don't like about yourself, know that you have the power to make positive personal changes. Accept yourself where you are and determine where you want to go, the benefits of going there, how to get started, and the steps you have to take.

It takes resolve, practice, and vigilance to come out of the shadows of deceit and deepen your commitment to truth. Give yourself the gift of patience to sustain you along the way and avoid discouragement.

Vow to no longer be a holder of secrets, yours or anyone else's. Let the truth set you free—free from lies that can enslave you. Live a life of integrity that allows you to be open, honest, and transparent.

CHAPTER 22

Stress Is Inevitable—Use It to Build Resilience

We are continually faced by great opportunities
brilliantly disguised as insoluble problems.
—Lee Iacocca

With the help of research, we are discovering how stress can exacerbate any health issue and perhaps even have a causal component. The initial reaction may be to wish that stress could be avoided by having a problem-free life. With this type of thinking, when a problem that "should not" have occurred does happen, you ruminate on the event, dwelling on how unlucky you are and how bad things are always happening to you. You fear that the demands are greater than your ability to meet those demands. You find yourself braced for the next shoe to drop, living a life of negative projection, complaining, and discontent.

The problem is not that there are problems. The
problem is expecting otherwise and thinking
that having problems is a problem.
—Isaac Rubin

However, since no one has ever had a stress-free life, the challenge becomes to build resilience to stressful situations by changing your perception of stress. Once you recognize that stress is inevitable and you change your approach to stress, one day you will be surprised that life simply does not *feel* so overwhelmingly stressful anymore. Old thinking was that riding a wave of adversity entitled you to future smooth sailing, and the next unexpected wave triggered justifiable outrage. With a change in perspective, you ride the first wave and apply what you learned to ride all the other waves you encounter. A positive attitude is a great asset in building resilience.

You learn to look back at the past with different eyes. You reflect on how you were able to work through each stressful event and validate your resourcefulness. Instead of a story of victimhood, it becomes a story of courage, and you record the strategies you used to forge forward. When others share stressful events in their lives, you focus on the steps they took to find solutions, and you thank them for sharing the experience with you. Thus you can learn without having to go through all these experiences yourself. Many who believe in a caring God and guardian angels rely on the following prayer:

> Either He will spare you from suffering or
> give you unfailing strength to bear it.
> —St. Francis de Sales

On the other hand, when you ruminate on your problems, the body *continuously* releases cortisol, and chronic elevated levels can have serious consequences. Too much cortisol can suppress the immune system, increase blood pressure and sugar, decrease libido, produce acne, and contribute to obesity and more. Research further indicates that the hormone cortisol, which is released during stress, can inhibit the formation of cells and decrease the gray matter in the hippocampus. As cortisol is linked with reducing the size of the hippocampus (memory, learning, and emotion), it is also linked with the increase and size and activity of the amygdala (fear responses and pleasure).

Simply put, for the caveman, the role of the amygdala was of vital importance; when there was a lion at the door, it was important to be able to spring into action. However, in our modern lives, if we carry the same chronic stress level as if the lion is always at the door, our brain will pay the price. When stress-arousing thoughts arise and there is no planning or action to be taken in the moment, then we can choose one thought over another by changing the channel, as we do when watching something undesirable on television.

"Ducks walk out of a lake, flap their wings and they fly off," says Sood. "When you face something stressful, particularly if it's not likely to repeat or doesn't have a huge long-term impact, you want to be able to shake it off and move on with life." When stress becomes simply a fact of life, you no longer feed the wolves of fear. "Why me?" is replaced with "Why not me?" This philosophy applies equally to feeling deserving of good things. You get in touch with the fact that all things are passing, the good and the bad. You remind yourself that you are resilient, courageous, vulnerable, positive, and curious. Living becomes so much more than simply staying alive. Your change in attitude takes you from surviving to thriving, a concept developed in workshops and seminars.

> "I read somewhere ... it is important in life
> not to be strong, but to feel strong.
> —Christopher McCandless

The above quote brought thoughts of my mother. Her steadfast faith kept her plowing forward no matter the odds, especially after the sudden, unexpected death of my father at the age of forty-two. As a young widow with four children back in the 1940s, she found creative ways to support her family. She identified the need for a movie theatre in the small town in which we lived. Despite huge obstacles, she qualified for the loans to finance the project and maneuvered through the pitfalls of new construction. The opening was a great success. Within a year, she was challenged by a large competing corporation that wanted to shut her down.

Had she stacked the mounting stressors—the untimely death of her husband, four children, no financial reserve, fear of failure, and being labeled irresponsible or crazy to risk everything—she might have buckled under the stress. Many sleepless nights were filled with tears and prayers. There were many twists and turns in this story, and the corporation ultimately offered to buy her out, providing a financial accomplishment quite unusual for a woman in those times. She never doubted that God was on her side. She also believed that her husband and parents were watching over her from heaven. She bravely faced each emotional and financial stressor and never doubted her inner strength based on her unswerving faith.

Applying an earlier tool of *not taking things personally* helps you see that problems happen to everyone, and you can learn from them. You stop stacking the problems, like boxes, one on top of the other, to create an insurmountable pile. You learn to compartmentalize, laying each box side by side, to prioritize and focus on one task at a time. This makes everything more manageable. Compartmentalizing also helps you separate which problems are yours to address and which ones are a part of someone else's journey. You explore options and take action on the areas within your control and allow the rest to unfold.

> Resilience is the strength and speed of our
> response to adversity—and we can build it.
> —Option B

A process for changing your relationship with stress is to bring your awareness to the stressful situation and observe it from different perspectives. Remind yourself that everything is impermanent, breathe in the helpful (whatever you learn), and breathe out the harmful (the suffering and stress). You learn to tolerate any negative emotions, touch them with compassion, and release them with your "this too will pass" philosophy.

Journaling your thoughts can increase insight, and shredding what you wrote is an effective way of releasing pent-up emotions. Sharing them with a trusted friend can be comforting and helpful. You incorporate stress relievers, such as meditation, prayer, exercise, yoga, dancing, and a host of others, following a suggestion for the activities to be equal and opposite to the stressor. A motivational speaker, whose stressful career involved airports, hotels, meeting rooms, sleep deprivation, and meals on the run, would take time out for outdoor, peaceful activities. He found he could shut off the hectic thoughts and immerse himself in the present moment, after which he would return refreshed and recharged to face the daily challenges again.

> Walking in nature or viewing pictures of nature improves
> people's ability to concentrate, focus and problem-solve.
> —Arbor Day Foundation

Humor can also be used to lighten the impact of a traumatic event. There were several articles written about how our fortieth president, Ronald Reagan, effectively used humor after the assassination attempt on March 30, 1981, by

John W. Hinkley Jr. Reagan was unaware at first that three others had been seriously wounded. He realized it was crucial to impart to the country that he was going to bounce back. He knew that his usual use of humor could get this message across, perhaps better than any other official reassurance.

According to *Time*'s coverage of the assassination attempt, the very first thing he said to the First Lady when she arrived at the hospital was, "Honey, I forgot to duck," a reference to a one-liner used by boxer Jack Dempsey. The magazine compiled a list of his best reactions to the shooting and his own injuries, one of which was directed to surgeons as he entered the operating room, "Please tell me you're Republicans."

> On particularly rough days, when I'm sure I
> can't possibly endure, I remind myself that my
> track record of getting through bad days so far
> is 100 percent, and that's pretty good.
> —Author unknown

Key Points

- Breathe.
- Honor your initial feelings.
- Explore the challenges from all perspectives.
- Use reframing to identify the hidden blessings.
- Compartmentalize rather than stack issues.
- Have a plan of action to address areas within your control.
- Use appropriate humor to lighten your heart.
- Learn and grow.
- Make peace your primary goal.

Thus, there are many healthy ways to accept and work through the inevitable stressors, rather than attempt to resist or ignore them or succumb to self-pity. Each event can be experienced as a growth opportunity, and you move on unencumbered by bitterness. Visualizing a positive outcome can be a great survival tool. Align yourself with problem-solvers to influence your perception of stress and build resilience. Simple strategies can interrupt the downward spiral of self-defeating thoughts. "I'm too blessed to be stressed" can create a quick turnaround to shift the focus to curiosity, learning, and appropriate action or nonaction.

CHAPTER 23

Self-Love, Self-Care

Taking care of myself is a big job. No
wonder I avoided it for so long.
—Anonymous

This chapter has two parts in order to first explore the topic, followed by practical information to motivate action.

Part I—Meaning and Understanding

There have been several interpretations of Jesus's response from the Bible in Matthew 22:36–40 (KJV):

> Master, which is the great commandment in the law? Jesus said unto him, Thou shalt love the Lord thy God with all thy heart, and with all thy soul, and with all thy mind. This is the first and great commandment. And the second is like unto it. Thou shalt love thy neighbor as thyself. On these two commandments hang all Law and the Prophets.

One could conclude that without self-love/self-compassion, you have nothing to offer others. A possible barrier is the confusion with ego and narcissism, which are the opposite of self-love. The person who is imprisoned by ego is constantly seeking to fulfil the ego's insatiable demands. Self-love, on the other hand, is loving, accepting, and appreciating yourself, which promotes well-being and makes you kinder to others.

Another barrier to self-love is the tyranny of perfectionism, where there is very low tolerance for mistakes. An error of any kind generates harsh, punitive self-talk, which can continue long after the event. Ruminating about what you "shoulda, coulda, woulda," done, which is exhausting and self-defeating, can be replaced with "next time" this is how you'll handle a similar situation better. You take the lighthearted approach that you are human, and life will always give you opportunities to practice imperfection.

I am careful not to confuse excellence with perfection.
Excellence, I can reach for; perfection is God's business.
—Michael J. Fox

So, what else may get in the way? Elsie's story shows how self-love can be eroded by unhealthy relationships. When others would tell her how pretty she looked, she could not see it. She could only hear her brother's critical, destructive words and the disapproval of her parents, who made it obvious that her brother was their favorite. She ultimately found the holistic approach, including therapy and prayer, to transcend the negativity with self-compassion and regain self-love. She went on to surround herself with positive people who helped her get in touch with her blessings.

For some, barriers to self-love begin in childhood, where the first messages were of being unwanted and undesirable. For example, the son who internalized his father's hurtful words, "Your name should be Waste Of Space," and the ridicule about his weight. Famous actor Marlon Brando wrote in his book that his father never had anything good to say about him. Despite his troubled youth, he went on to be nominated for eight Academy Awards and won his first Oscar in 1955 for his role in *On the Waterfront*.

> Your task is not to seek for love, but merely
> to seek and find all the barriers within
> yourself that you have built against it.
> —Rumi

Removing barriers to self-love begins with coming to terms with how you truly feel about yourself. If for some reason you dislike me, that's unfortunate; if I dislike me, that's unbearable! Self-acceptance and self-compassion foster self-love by opening the path to identifying your strengths and flaws without judgment. Energy is channeled toward personal growth.

Compare the impact of early negative messages to the following tale. The source is purportedly from Tolba Phanem, African poet. Although the authenticity has been challenged, this story carries a beautiful, uplifting message worth sharing.

> When a woman of a certain African tribe knows she is pregnant, she goes into the jungle with other women, and together they connect with nature, pray and meditate until they find The Song of the Child. They return to the tribe and teach it to everyone else.
>
> As the child develops in the mother's womb, she sings this song to the unborn child. When the child is born and at every birthday celebration, the villagers get together and sing the child's song. When the child begins his education, community comes together to hear

the child sing his own song. When it comes to his wedding, he hears his song again. Finally, when his soul is leaving this world, family and friends gather around him, and like at his birth, sing his song to accompany him on the final journey.

Create your own song to validate your strengths and replace any destructive messages you may have been subjected to. Gain an understanding of the reason you think and subsequently feel the way you do. Be encouraged that you can become your best self. Today, commit to treating yourself like someone you love.

Self-care is often misconstrued as selfishness, and there is a simple distinction between the two. A selfish act would come from a person who simply does not care about anyone else. Obviously, that is not true for you. Self-care, on the other hand, is the interconnected approach to taking care of your emotional, physical, and spiritual well-being. This equips you to build a better relationship with self and others.

The importance of self-care is often illustrated in this airplane analogy from in-flight instructions. You are directed, in the event of an emergency, to place the oxygen mask over your own face first before assisting others. You certainly cannot help anyone if you pass out from lack of oxygen. Another humorous analogy is recognizing that if you are a tow truck, you must fix your own flat tire first before you can tow other vehicles. How many times have you heard the expression "Physician, heal thyself!"

Giving and receiving are the two wings of generosity. You cannot be a true giver if you block your ability to receive, because that type of giving often comes with control and expectations. Healthy giving is a simple act of kindness, and there is no attachment or resentment. Healthy receiving opens the way to expressing gratitude and blessing the giver. When you believe that "what I give to you I give to myself," giving and receiving become effortless. Like the clear pond, there is an inflow and an outflow. Without an inflow, the pond would dry up, and without an outflow, the pond would become stagnant and overflow the banks. So, catch yourself when you fall back into thinking your healthy actions are "selfish" and replace this with the appropriate word, "self-care."

Part II—Method and Motivation

The World Health Organization gives this definition: "Health is a state of complete mental, physical and social well-being and not merely the absence of disease or infirmity." Many wellness experts have embraced Dr. James Chestnut's revolutionary concept of wellness, which is adapted here to simplify and motivate lifestyle changes. Here is a handy formula that you could use: TW + EW + MW + SW = BW (Think Well + Eat Well + Move Well + Sleep Well = Be Well).

Think well—TW. Observe every thought and make the conscious effort to reinforce only the thoughts that strengthen you. Learn to navigate challenges such as stress/anxiety, fatigue, overscheduling/multitasking, and depression/mood problems. Retrain your brain and enhance inner peace through reading, study, mindfulness, meditation, and spiritual pursuits. Let destructive thoughts drift away like a leaf floating down the river. The positive thoughts you create have far-reaching effects. How you think about things affects how you feel and influences your day-to-day experiences.

> Age is a question of mind over matter. If
> you don't mind, it doesn't matter.
> —Hall of Fame pitcher, Satchel Paige

Cultures that respect and revere their elders regard aging as wisdom and a great resource. Other cultures that have a negative view of aging can be dismissive and impatient, thereby setting themselves up for future unhappiness as they go through the inevitable aging process. A wonderful woman known as Peace Pilgrim was asked, "How is it that you are so vital and seem so happy in your old age?" Her response was "I don't eat any junk food, and I don't have any junk thoughts." This is a great segue to the next topic.

> The secret to all disease is in your gut.
> —Hippocrates

Eat well—EW. In the old days, young ladies were often counseled that "the way to a man's heart is through his stomach," an amusing way of suggesting that a woman could make a man love her by cooking good meals. Today, these words have significant meaning. "The way to the heart is through the stomach" elevates the importance of proper nutrition to maintain health for longevity and prevent disease. Become vigilant of all the things you allow into your body.

When you make the conscious effort to maintain a healthy diet, you enjoy this new way of eating. You avoid and ultimately lose the desire for unhealthy items such as refined sugar and carbs, excessive alcohol or toxic drugs, and foods with harmful preservatives. Then, there is no need to go on a diet, because you have changed your relationship with food by consuming whole natural foods for nourishment. Current research, including work by Dr. Donald Layman, Professor Emeritus, University of Illinois, indicates the importance of optimizing protein in your daily meals, along with other recommendations, such as enzymes for proper absorption and the importance of cleansing.

Follow the recommendation for water intake. The amount

of water in the human body ranges from 50–75 percent. Blood is mostly water, and our muscles, lungs, and brain all contain a lot of water. Water is needed to regulate body temperature and to provide the means for nutrients to travel to all our organs. Water also transports oxygen to our cells, removes waste, and protects our joints and organs. A few of the many symptoms of dehydration are dry mouth and eyes, headaches, palpitations, decreased urine output, bad breath, and muscle cramps. Begin and end your day with a glass of water and have six more glasses throughout the day. In fact, look up the program Japanese Water Therapy, which advises to drink three glasses of water (twenty-two ounces) upon arising, brush the teeth afterward, and wait forty-five minutes before eating anything.

Move well—MW. Ongoing studies are looking at the positive effects of exercise and good posture in slowing down muscle mass loss, which had formerly been seen as the inevitable result of aging. In addition to the exercises specifically recommended for sarcopenia (muscle mass loss), you can take better care of your physical body by simple steps like walking. Others have found yoga or Pilates helpful, or fun activities like Zumba and aerobics.

You also get social support by joining a gym or having a trainer. Insurance companies recognize that providing free exercise classes for seniors through local gyms is a good investment. In an article by Stephanie Watson, it states, "Exercise, one of the best ways to protect your intellect, sends a surge of blood and oxygen to nourish brain cells and it prevents brain shrinkage with age."

A great example of mental and physical activity is ballroom dancing, which is enjoyed by folks well into their eighties and nineties. They get the physical exercise from the actual movement and posture, while the brain is stimulated in recording the various steps in time with the music. There is also the social aspect of the synergy with other dancers as they all move around the floor.

An even bigger surprise was that regularly engaging in social dancing lowered the seniors' risk of dementia by a staggering 76 percent. Neurologist Dr. Joe Verghese at Albert Einstein College of Medicine followed elderly subjects over an impressive twenty-one year period. The theory proposed by Dr. Verghese and his fellow researchers is that social dance is an activity that activates and takes advantage of our brains' neuroplasticity. Neuroplasticity refers to the brain's ability to change and grow through life. This occurs whenever something new is learned. The brain never stops changing through learning.

Ballroom dance and other forms that involve cooperation between two partners, leading and following special steps and improvising, involves quick decision-making that creates new neural pathways. More pathways provide more accessibility to the stored information, and the less likely you are to forget it.

Kendall Dance Studio in Miami has students of all ages, from kids to seniors. These are encouraging examples. Margaret Enciso enjoyed an active lifestyle until increasing hip pain began to threaten her quality of life. She weighed the options and proceeded with hip surgery. Her positive attitude and desire to return to dancing as soon as possible fueled her rehabilitative physical therapy. In record time, she was back to the mental, physical, and social activity of ballroom dancing, feeling fortunate and grateful. Dr. William (Bill) Jackson had a consistent routine of walking and working out at the gym. After retirement, he looked for a hobby he could be passionate about. Ballroom dancing gave him the mind/body/spirit stimulation he desired and was the perfect complement to his exercise program. Pearl Daniels Vann, a feisty lady who is still ballroom dancing at age ninety-seven, receives an enthusiastic welcome at the studio parties and other social events. She added physical therapy to her regime and gained improved balance and posture.

Interestingly enough, there is another important factor. Current research is looking at the harmful effects of sitting for prolonged periods. The human body is built to be active and moving all day. While periods of rest are necessary, too much sitting time, for example TV and computer time, and times sitting in automobiles, is linked to a host of at least twenty-four chronic diseases and conditions and increases premature mortality risk. The body with its 360 joints and seven hundred skeletal muscles is built for movement. The recommendation is to sit straight and get up and move around every half an hour.

A new study from Harvard suggests that inactivity can be as hazardous to your health as smoking and that a sedentary lifestyle is the cause of one in ten deaths worldwide. Levine is credited with the saying, "Sitting is the new smoking."

Sleep well—SW. Most people feel better after a good night's sleep. Studies have indicated that most adults operate best on seven to eight hours of quality sleep on a regular basis. Teens and younger children need more. Adequate sleep is an important component of a healthy lifestyle. There is mounting evidence that adequate sleep is essential for memory and learning. Insufficient sleep impacts your motivation, judgment, perception, and mood. In a 2011 review article, Richard Stickgold and Erin Wamsley explained, "During all stages of sleep, the mind and brain are working to process new memories, consolidating them into long-term storage and integrating recently acquired information with past experience."

Sleep deprivation is a precursor to many problems. Lowered performance, decreased alertness, and daytime sleepiness impair your ability to think and process and retain information. Other ramifications include injuries at work and automobile injuries: drowsy driving has been responsible for at least 100,000 automobile crashes, 71,000 injuries, and 1,550 fatalities each year, as estimated by the National Highway Traffic Safety Administration. Additionally, you are probably not much fun to be around when you are tired and irritable, so your relationships suffer too. Napoleon Bonaparte is said to have slept about four hours per night because of his stressful lifestyle, and contemporaries felt that sleep deprivation could have compromised his decision-making and contributed to his loss at Waterloo.

The recommendations given in "sleep hygiene" provide helpful tips, such as going to bed and arising about the same time each day. My old habit of late nights during the week and trying to catch up on sleep over the weekend did not work. By Sunday night, I would be so rested that I would get to bed really late and start the cycle all over again. I used the preceding tip to begin the process of changing my sleep pattern.

It is also helpful to create a peaceful nighttime ritual, such as pleasant music or quiet meditation to train your body to respond to signals that you are preparing to go to bed. That of course means not watching the news and any other arousing shows right before bed. According to sleep.org, "The blue light emitted by screens on cell phones, computers, tablets, and televisions restrain the production of melatonin, the hormone that controls your sleep/wake cycle or circadian rhythm. Reducing melatonin makes it harder to fall and stay asleep. Give yourself at least 30 minutes of gadget-free transition time before hitting the hay. Even better: Make your bedroom a technology-free zone—keep your electronics outside the room (that includes a TV!)." Another important caution is limiting your alcohol/caffeine and fluid intake at bedtime.

Hopefully, this is just enough information to motivate you to review the wealth of articles available and follow through on sleep hygiene recommendations to see how they work for you. Most importantly, you can break your dependence on sleep medication.

Be well—BW: the sum of the parts. Live, thrive, and be healthy! A moment-to-moment commitment to wellness, self-care, and self-compassion incorporates mind, body, and spirit. All thoughts, feelings, and actions impact all areas. When these are congruent, there is harmony and well-being. Life provides constant distractions that can interrupt mindfulness and disturb your equanimity. These distractions are simply a part of the tapestry of life, and as such, you can pause, observe, process, learn, and release to regain the inner calm that makes self-care and self-compassion possible. As Jack LaLane's widow, Elaine, explained, "It's not what you do some of the time that counts, it's what you do most of the time."

> The body is like a child. It needs constant prompting and
> training and discipline and praise and appreciation. Your
> body needs your attention, your love, your training …
> Look at that wonderful body temple. It is precious to you.
> —Myrtle Fillmore

George Vaillant (Vaillant 2002), who heads the most extensive longitudinal study of human development, has found that as we mature and age, we are less influenced by our early experiences and much more affected by our choices, attitudes, and actions. We can go on to rewrite our ongoing autobiography.

Key Points

- Breathe.
- Adapt the formula TW + EW + MW + SW = BW for self-care and well-being (Think Well + Eat Well + Move Well + Sleep Well = Be Well).
- Practice self-compassion and compassion for others.
- Choose positive friends.
- Give and receive helpful support.
- Be your own best friend.

Be inspired to reflect on your lifestyle. Strive for a healthy balance. Recognize how self-care enhances your connectedness with humanity. Assimilate and apply helpful messages. When you focus on the inner goodness of self and others, life becomes meaningful.

CHAPTER 24

Give Only What You Want to Receive

I have found that if you love life, life will love you back.
—Arthur Rubenstein

Give only what you want to receive; if you want respect, give respect. Same with love, kindness, acceptance, and more. The way you treat others sends a message to the universe that this is the way you want to be treated. Thus, you can identify, consider, and change your undesirable behaviors. Giving and receiving are the two wings of generosity. When you give to others only what you would happily receive, you feel blessed.

Words from the song "Nature Boy" are "The greatest thing you'll ever learn, is just to love and be loved in return." Chances are most people would agree with that sentiment and would like to be in a loving relationship. This gives you the opportunity to ask yourself, "Would I like to be in a relationship with someone exactly like me?" If you want to be loved, it would follow that you need to be lovable. With honest self-evaluation, do you think that others feel safe and comfortable around you? You reflect on what it would be like to be on the receiving end of your words and actions. Whatever your circumstances might have been, you can commit to getting better, not bitter. You can work on identifying the barriers to getting all that you desire and learn to be open and receptive to all the good. You embrace the golden rule and do unto to others as you would have others do unto you.

> The only way to have a friend is to be one.
> —Ralph Waldo Emerson

This becomes clearer when you adopt the principles of Namaste, an ancient Sanskrit greeting still in everyday use in India and especially on the trail in the Nepal Himalaya. "I honor the place in you of light, of love, of truth, of peace; I honor the place in you where if you and I are in that place then there is only one of us." How might your relationships be influenced if this became your daily greeting and you really believed that we are all one? This would certainly foster the gentler, kinder world that you desire.

Consider the concept of respect. People often say that they want to be respected yet withhold respect from someone they deem unworthy. If you pick and choose to whom you will offer respect, then you are not giving consistently what you want to receive. The homeless person under the bridge is as deserving of respect as anyone else, because inside that person lives a core of goodness, and you do not know that person's circumstances. Perhaps one respectful word from you could be a turning point in that person's life. Through the eyes of compassion, you will see yourself in that other person and be grateful for the blessings in your own life.

Here's one version of this often-told little parable. A man moved to a new town. He asked a local resident whether the people there were friendly or not.

The resident asked the man, "What were people like where you used to live?"

The newcomer scowled and said, "They were really an unfriendly and rude bunch, and I couldn't wait to get away from that place."

The resident said, "Well, I'm afraid you'll find the people here are pretty much the same."

A week later, another man came to town. He happened to meet the same resident and asked him the same question about the people in that town. The local resident asked this second newcomer the same question: "What were the people like in the town where you used to live?"

This newcomer smiled and said, "Oh, that town was the friendliest place you could ever imagine."

The local returned the smile and said, "Well, I'm glad to hear it. I think you'll find people here are very friendly too."

What if these visitors made the commitment to give only what they wanted to receive from the people of that town? How might their experience be affected?

Do you think you can do your part to make this world a friendly place? Your answer to this important question will greatly influence your day-to-day experience of living. You can look for the highest good in yourself as you look for the highest good in each person. You can choose to operate from a source of positive energy.

This story shows that, with any behavior, you have to claim it to change it. Jolene had grown up in an environment where there was neglect, abuse, and abandonment. Through sheer determination, she made it through college and into a successful career. It was no surprise that she went from one dysfunctional relationship to another. Feeling discouraged, she stopped dating for a while until she met Arnold. After a short courtship with Arnold, she discovered that she was pregnant. They discussed it and decided they would move in together. Fear and lack of trust kept her emotionally distant, and she felt justified in her intermittent explosive behaviors. Occasionally, her emotional void would become overwhelming, and she would reach out to Arnold for support. Over time, Arnold became so wary of her erratic behaviors that he disengaged for self-protection and could not meet her needs.

The vicious cycle continued until Jolene's escalating alcohol use propelled her into treatment. There she was able to face her demons and take a nonblaming look at her destructive pattern of behavior. Meanwhile, Arnold began his own process of therapy to discover how his past had influenced his choosing this relationship and what personal changes he needed to make. For the first time, each felt encouraged that personal change and growth could open up the possibility of a healthy relationship of mutual giving and receiving.

> To love is to recognize yourself in another.
> —Eckhart Tolle

Validate positive changes. Don't miss an opportunity to compliment, praise, and encourage. We have learned that unexpressed love is the greatest cause of our sorrow and regrets. Sometimes we wait until someone dies to express their value in our lives. This often begins in childhood. A child who is well behaved and easygoing is likely to get far less attention than the child who is prone to temper tantrums and defiance. The child learns that they can usually get their parents' attention with acting-out behaviors. This can become an unconscious game. You reverse the process when you give your attention to the smallest positive changes, creating an environment of appreciation and growth.

> Conquer the devils with a little thing called love.
> —Bob Marley

When we witness the heartless, despicable deeds of people like Kim Jong Un or followers of Isis, this horror can propel us to do the complete *opposite*. With a commitment to consciously engage in acts of kindness and compassion, each action can produce a positive ripple effect flowing outward to the whole world. Mother Teresa is said to have advised us to begin each day with a smile and say yes, knowing that not all of us can do great things, but we can do small things with great love.

Become part of the collective energy to reflect these lyrics: "What the world needs now, is love, sweet love, that's the only thing there's much too little of." You incorporate the philosophy that "what I give to you, I give to myself." This belief frees you from any attachment or expectations. Others on your path help you at the right time. This keeps you thankful that you can give or receive effortlessly.

Key Points

- Breathe.
- Identify what you would like to receive in life and in all your relationships.
- Evaluate your actions to determine which ones to reinforce and which to change.
- Be patient and persevere, knowing that change takes time.
- Validate positive changes, yours and others.
- Contribute to the collective energy.

Take the time to clarify your desires. Honestly evaluate your own actions. Determine if what you do aligns with what you want. Become the best you and invite the best in others. Revisit any missteps and return to the right path. Contemplate this question: what would the world be like if everyone behaved exactly the way you do?

CHAPTER 25

Renew Your Happiness Every Day

*Don't wait for things to get easier, simpler, better.
Life will always be complicated. Learn to be happy
right now. Otherwise you'll run out of time.*
—Unknown

Chances are most people would say that they really want to be happy. Yet when asked, "Are you happy?" they might hesitate to respond, because they are consciously or unconsciously waiting for specific things to happen before they can be happy. "I'll be happy when ..." may mean "when I have this or that" or "when you do this or that."

Happiness can become even more elusive. Eve lived in the Garden of Eden, filled with delicious fruits. When she shifted her desire to the one fruit that was forbidden, she made that become the measure of her happiness, and she lost sight of all that she had.

*It isn't what you have or who you are or where you
are or what you are doing that makes you happy
or unhappy. It is what you think about it.*
—Dale Carnegie

Research reveals that happy people view problems as temporary, impersonal, and solvable. This belief is empowering because it makes everything feel manageable.

Happiness is more of a mind-set than a mood—being happy versus feeling happy. Immediate negative thoughts are observed and challenged. Happy people associate happiness with resilience, optimism, and growth. After analyzing and understanding the problem, they identify the appropriate course of action.

> Most folks are about as happy as they
> make up their minds to be.
> —Abe Lincoln

This story shows the importance of not delaying happiness. Dev had lived in an unhappy marriage for more than thirty years. As her husband's alcoholism progressed, it began to take a heavier toll on her and their children. She felt stuck, wanting her husband to stop drinking so they could live a normal life. Each time he told her he was ready to stop, she would feel relieved that finally they could be happy.

After multiple disappointments from her husband's inability to keep his word, Dev could no longer appreciate the periods when he avoided alcohol. She found herself fearful of the next episode of uncontrolled drinking and distressing behaviors.

The escalating consequences prompted Dev's husband to finally commit to going to treatment, and he seemed motivated to deal with this formidable problem. After failed attempts there and at subsequent treatment programs, he seemed to give up. Dev confided to her support group, "I can't stand feeling helpless. I always think there must be something I could do, but sometimes, of course, there's nothing."

Dev posed a question in despair one day, "How much

longer will he continue to live like this?" She was unprepared for the response she received, "How much longer will *you* continue to live like this? Don't let misery be the story of your life." That was Dev's moment of clarity. She realized that she could not keep waiting for her husband's actions to make her happy. She had to take the steps to generate her own happiness.

> Be happy for this moment. This moment is your life.
> —Omar Khayyam

Dev reflected on the theme song from a serious, sad, and humorous play, "Even when your life's falling apart, you can still have a really good day." She began slowly to take care of herself. Overcoming her apprehension, she made her first trip alone to visit relatives in another state. Despite multiple phone calls from her husband, she enjoyed the visit. This opened a new door for her, and she began to find joy in the simplest of things.

Dev kept her hope alive that her husband would find life-giving sobriety, but she would no longer put her own life on hold. This helped her let go of her anger and resentment from all the years of futile efforts to get him to change. She realized that he might fall into the category of alcoholics who were not able to overcome this repetition compulsion. As she witnessed the decline of his quality of life, she knew in her heart that she would not leave him. She had to find the way to support him and be happy with the other positive aspects of her life.

When complications from his alcoholism took his life, Dev was able to accept her sadness at the loss, and she hoped that he had finally found peace. She could look back on their life together and not have to blame him for her unhappiness or harbor resentment. When she aligned with the Buddhist philosophy that suffering comes from wanting things to be different, Dev was ready to make room for happiness by letting go of misery. She made the decision to identify and release any blocks to her happiness.

> The first to apologize is the bravest. The
> first to forgive is the strongest.
> The first to forget is the happiest.
> —David Voth

There are also people who have a huge barrier to overcome—the irrational fear that if you let go and be happy, something awful will happen. This is a condition known as Cherophobia, from the Greek word *chairo*, which means "I rejoice." Some medical experts consider this to be a form of anxiety. Anything fun has to be too good to be true. Thus, there is a reluctance to do anything that could bring happiness, and they become accustomed to unhappiness.

Apprehension can sometimes be the result of childhood experiences, where a happy event was followed right away by punishment or tragedy. In the past there may have been little tolerance for "wasting time" or having fun, without fear of negative consequences.

Therapy can help people work through fear from past trauma or conflict and find the way to balance. They learn how to apply appropriate caution to replace the ominous fear that blocks happiness. They arrive at a sense of well-being through guidance and practice, including being happy for others.

What if you were to change your perception and make a vow to unconditional happiness? Happiness is renewable and requires regular conscious effort. Constant reminders that happiness is a choice and happiness is an inside job can set the compass for navigating your journey. Habit is described as an automatic response created by the brain to make things better. You could make a daily habit of renewing your vow to unconditional happiness by making your to-be list (before you make your to-do list). "Today I will be happy" could head the list.

When challenges arise, as they will, you would activate your curiosity by asking, "What can I learn from this?" Thus you gain insight and incorporate the lesson. You could expand your daily affirmation, "Today I will be happy for no reason."

> In the long run the pessimist may be proved right, but
> the optimist will have a better time on the trip.
> —Daniel Reardon

Happiness comes from our choices, not from our circumstances. Consider people having a shared experience on vacation. One person is intrigued by the unique differences in the environment and culture, while the other person complains about the discomfort of things not being the way they are at home. Imagine how our day-to-day experience of life could be enhanced by understanding that happiness is a way of thinking and being. Positive thoughts become the stimulus for positive emotions.

There is a Zen story about a student who went to his meditation teacher and said, "My meditation is horrible! I feel so distracted, or my legs ache, or I'm constantly falling asleep. It's just horrible!"

"Don't worry. It will pass," the teacher said matter-of-factly.

A week later, the student came back to his teacher. "My meditation is wonderful! I feel so aware, so peaceful, so alive! It's just wonderful!"

The teacher replied matter-of-factly, "Don't worry. It will pass."

Werner Heisenberg was awarded the Nobel Peace Prize

for Physics in 1932. He is best known for his uncertainty principle and theory of quantum mechanics, which he published at the age of twenty-three in 1925. Heisenberg's contribution that "We live in eternal uncertainty" can elevate the importance of choosing happiness without regard for outside events.

Consider these simple activities to boost your happiness, along with others you learn from many sources. Take a little time out to access a reservoir of happy memories as a reminder that everything passes. Talk about happy times with friends and cherish every positive experience. Laugh at some jokes, smile often, and sing in the shower. Pray or meditate. Redefine age. Researchers found that happiness may slow aging and improve health. Fill your bubble of happiness with positive thoughts every day and don't allow anyone to burst your bubble.

> If we cannot be Happy in spite of our difficulties,
> what good is our spiritual practice?
> —Maha Ghosananda

Key Points

- Breathe.
- Acknowledge that happiness is an inside job.
- Identify what is blocking your happiness and commit to removing these blocks.
- Adopt many techniques to reinforce happiness every day.
- Let your happiness come from your choices, not your circumstances.
- Smile and brighten up the world.

Give yourself a break and renew your happiness every day. It is easy to be distracted by events and succumb to negative emotions. Take any necessary action to return to the mind-set of happiness. Everything is temporary, so enjoy the good times and reflect on them to help you through challenging times. Ten years from now, these will be the good old days. Be happy now!

CHAPTER 26

Focus on What You Want to Attract—Law of Attraction

If you believe it will work out, you'll see opportunities.
If you believe it won't you will see obstacles.
—Wayne Dyer

The law of attraction is one of the most powerful universal laws. A simple definition is the ability to attract into your life what you focus on. In every moment, you are sending out thoughts and attracting negative or positive experiences accordingly. Instead of bracing for catastrophe, you can plan for abundance. When you understand and accept responsibility that the things you put your attention to are the things you end up attracting, you develop a persistent, patient, positive process (PPPP) of creating the vision and taking action.

Spend more time smiling than frowning, and
more time praising than criticizing.
—Richard Branson

Recognize how unguarded thoughts shape your future and identify what is blocking your path to the life you want to manifest. Complaining and criticizing have been compared to evil twins who seek to entangle you in a web of discontent.

Complaining hijacks your focus and keeps you going around in circles as you envy others and feel inadequate by comparison. You vacillate between pride in your accomplishments and despair that you have not achieved enough.

Indecision delays action, which in turn creates more anxiety. It keeps you stuck in the belief that *I'm running out of time; I'm not where I should be.* This mental noise can suffocate your dream and create distress. Dale Carnegie offered similar advice: "Don't criticize, condemn or complain," all of which keeps your attention on what you don't want. Complaining is nonacceptance of the present moment.

Often people will have a laundry list of all the things they do not want yet have no clear picture of what they want. With this in mind, you can explore what you would like, for example, in a relationship, and then be open to hearing what the other person finds important. Then you can determine what changes you are willing to make for personal growth and to strengthen the relationship. This redirects the attention to affirming thoughts and actions, and you can validate any positive change in yourself and the other person along the way. It behooves you to be mindful and vigilant about the thoughts that you replay and reinforce.

> All that we are is the result of what we have
> thought. The mind is everything.
> What we think we become.
> —Maharishi Mahesh Yogi

Anyone who saw the video or read the book *The Secret* received an effective presentation of the message that has been given over the centuries, from sources such as the Bible, "Ask and ye shall receive, seek and ye shall find, knock and it shall be opened unto thee," to Claude Bristol's *The Magic of Believing* and so many others. The message is timeless, and you have the choice to recognize the power of the law of attraction and focus on what you want to attract. Consider where you are now and how your thoughts, feelings, and actions guide your journey. A blind person asked St. Anthony, "Can there be anything worse than losing eyesight?" He replied, "Yes, losing your vision."

What is this vision we hear about, and how does vision relate to purpose and mission? There are many definitions of these concepts, and writing this book could serve as a concrete example. The purpose is to engage people by presenting ideas to affirm the importance of positive thinking and being kind and peaceful. My mission became to actually write this book. My vision is a world where people approach all things with a curious, compassionate heart, and love rules a peaceful world. Mahatma Gandhi invited us to become the change we want to see in the world. Hopefully this book will echo this message and become another drop in the ocean of loving connection. It would be awesome if you would also envision peace in all hearts.

By perseverance, the snail reached the ark.
—Charles Spurgeon

My mother was my first role model for the power of positive thinking. There were countless events where she found herself in very challenging situations, and each time she kept her faith with one of her favorite mantras, "With God, all things are possible." Once she had identified a goal, she would move in that direction, undeterred by obstacles. In 1980, my mother was seventy-seven years old. She decided that if she was going to fulfil a lifelong dream to see *The Passion Play* in Oberammergau, she would have to go that year, because this event took place every ten years.

She was fascinated by the story of the origin of this play.

In 1632, after nearly a quarter of the village died from the plague, the villagers prayed that God would have mercy and free the village from this sickness. They made a vow that the devout would present the passion of Christ Jesus in drama form every ten years. There were no further deaths, and the people of Oberammergau have kept their vow and missed only a couple of years during wars. The play was first performed in 1634 in Oberammergau, Bavaria, Germany, and covers the short final period of the life of Jesus, from his visit to Jerusalem to his crucifixion. Gifted poets set the play to verse, and performers must be native Oberammergauers, amateurs, and persons of high morals. Villagers begin a year ahead to grow their hair, and the hundreds of actors consider this a labor of love and receive no pay for their time and effort. The productions run for seven hours, with a break for lunch, four days a week for five months.

With about ten days to put this trip together and procure tickets, this seemed like an impossible task. Only one tour company in New York still had tickets, which were sold as part of an extensive tour. Undeterred, my mother said, "We will go and get the tickets there." My unspoken thoughts were, *Yeah right, just like that!*

We took off for Munich on September 25, having been warned that accommodation in Oberammergau and tickets to the performance were sold out. When we landed in Munich, our lost luggage was tracked to the connecting city of Frankfurt. There were three more flights that day from Frankfurt, and the hope was that our luggage would be on one of them. I left my mother in the company of other passengers with the same problem and went in search of tickets.

There were small, empty booths at the airport advertising *Oberammergau Passion Play*. I finally located one with staff and inquired about tickets. The agent looked at me in disbelief, reminding me that there were only two performances left, and they had been sold out for two years. As I just stood there gathering my thoughts, the other agent rushed out and said that a couple had canceled their reservation and turned in their package just an hour earlier. This included two nights' accommodation and tickets to the play. Payment had to be by cash, and there was no way to verify if these were legitimate tickets. With much apprehension, I gave them the cash, received the vouchers to present to the local tour company, and hoped for the best. I shared my concerns with my mother, and she assured me that this was all in divine order.

Our bags were the last two to come off the final flight of the day from Frankfurt. We got to our hotel and had a nice dinner. After our hot showers, we climbed into bed feeling exhausted and hopeful. That night, a half an hour from our hotel, the Oktoberfest bombing by terrorists killed thirteen people and injured 211. Unaware of this tragedy, the next morning, after a hearty breakfast, we set off on a pleasant drive through the picturesque Bavarian countryside to Oberammergau. We went directly to the local tour company and exchanged our voucher for the package. We sat in awe for a few minutes and said a prayer of gratitude and relief.

The next and final day of the performance, September 28, we arrived at the theater that has a seating capacity for more than 4,500 people and discovered that our seats were perfectly situated in the center, five rows from the stage. My mother had received her miracle, which she had never doubted. We took a deep breath and whispered, "Thank you, Lord."

If you must fast-forward to the future, rather than project negative, project positive. This, of course, keeps you headed in the right direction, turning stumbling blocks into stepping-stones.

Sometimes you win, sometimes you learn.
Take the first step.
—Unknown

A recommendation for inviting abundance is to create a vision board. The simplest version is to get a peg board and place this where you can see it at least once per day. Identify what you would like to invite into your life. Place notes on the board, or be more creative and cut out pictures or symbols to go along with the words. Add a notation of "thank you" each time something on your vision board manifests. This becomes a daily validation of your dreams and a reminder not to block your blessings because of discouraging words from negative self-talk or from others. Somewhat like the song from the movie *South Pacific*, "You got to have a dream. If you don't have a dream, how you gonna have a dream come true?"

Another recollection of the power of positive thinking is this story. My parents would take leisurely strolls through the neighborhood when my mother was pregnant with their second child. They often passed a house that was particularly appealing to my father, because it had been built by a retired sea captain and faced the ocean like a stationary ship. My father said wistfully, "Wouldn't it be great to own that home," immediately followed by, "Of course, it would never be possible for us." My mother's response was "Why not?" She lived in the land of possibility. My father simply gave a little shrug as they quietly continued their walk.

Twenty years later, we moved into that home. My mother looked out the window and felt the joy and the poignant sadness of owning this beautiful home—joy because of the incredible accomplishment, sadness because my father was not there to enjoy the blessing. He had died eight years earlier at age forty-two because of a medical misdiagnosis. It would take much more than a few chapters to share all the challenges she had to overcome as a single mother with four children during those times. Even at the darkest moments, she worked tirelessly and held fast to her faith.

> To accomplish great things, we must not only act,
> but also dream, not only plan, but also believe.
> —Anatole France

When you believe that your thoughts are magnets, you will be very vigilant about the thoughts you retain and the ones you dismiss. Focusing on what you want to attract means witnessing and letting go of self-imposed barriers and thoughts of being nondeserving of the good.

Approaching a final examination can be a setup for sabotaging success. An example would be procrastinating on completing assignments and being ill-prepared for the test, and later taking consolation in the fact that you are smart and would have passed if you had worked harder. Another flawed thinking is being afraid to study too hard because failure would then mean you are not too bright. In either case, failure is the expected result to further erode self-worth.

A shift in consciousness has to take place to break the pattern of self-defeating thoughts and behaviors. This begins with redefining failure. You realize that winners might actually have more losses along the way, compared to nonachievers. Failure becomes an indication that you discovered a method that did not work, and you learn from it. If Thomas Edison had been discouraged by failure, we might still be living in darkness. He is quoted as having said, "I have not failed. I've just found ten thousand ways that won't work."

Connect with and learn from achievers who have similar goals. Respect their dedication and celebrate their accomplishments. Banish jealousy, envy, discouragement, and insecurity, which block your path to success. See these leaders as your role models and be genuinely happy that they are doing well. Be confident that you too are on the way to accomplishing your dreams.

I may not be there yet, but I'm closer than I was yesterday.
—José N. Harris

The blade of grass that slowly pushes through the cement pathway can illustrate your power to accomplish your dreams. You were the winner of your very first competition. You may not have been the strongest or the fastest, yet you triumphed over three hundred million other competing sperm cells by completing the six-inch journey to the fertilized finish. Then the competition was over. With that type of determination and focus, clearly you are unique and have limitless potential.

The following questionnaire, which was handed out at a workshop, can stimulate curiosity and meaningful answers. You can pause here and reflect on these questions or return later.

- Does it give me life?
- Does it align with my core values?
- Does it require me to grow?
- Does it require the help of a higher power?
- Does it have good in it for others?

Begin the process of adopting positive thoughts. Firmly ask, believe, take action, and gratefully receive. Ask in faith for this or something better for the highest good of all concerned, and be open and receptive. Believe you deserve the fruits of your labor, as does everyone. Identify what action you must take and then take it. Discover the power of "yet";

if you have not achieved your dream, this simply means you haven't achieved your dream *yet*.

You'll see it When you believe it.
—Wayne Dyer

You can deepen your understanding of the power of your beliefs by exploring research on the role of the reticular activating system (RAS). The reticular activating system is a bundle of nerves at the base of the skull, and one of its functions is to act like a gatekeeper or filter in terms of what you hear and what goes into the subconscious. The subconscious is in a constant state of receiving.

The RAS uses your beliefs to create your reality. It keeps the focus on what it is already looking for and screens out everything else. This means you need to be very mindful what you focus on most, because your RAS will show you things to prove that this is true. If you say, "I'm not confident," or "I'll never have enough money," you are placing your focus on what you do not want. When you set your RAS to look for positives with self-talk, "I am confident," or "I'm good with money," then your RAS will start to show you things to prove that your new belief is true for you. Therefore, when you change the filter the RAS is using, things are different. Billy lamented, "I am so poor." His mother redirected him, "Don't ever say you are poor. Say you are having a temporary cash flow problem!"

Many articles on the RAS use the example of a time when you are planning to purchase a new car and you decide that you would like, for example, a silver Lexus. Suddenly you see a disproportionate number of silver Lexus cars on the road, whereas you had not noticed these cars a day earlier. When you invested your time and attention, your RAS was set to show you the particular car you were looking for.

It is imperative to ask the right questions. If you ask yourself, "Why can I never find a good-paying job with nice people?" your RAS will seek out the reasons why you cannot find the job you desire. The better question is, "What do I need to do to find the fulfilling job I want?" Your RAS will be set to achieve your goal, and you can take action. The more clear and tangible your desires are, the better your RAS will work for you. Some people say that they achieve what they put out to the universe. That is the RAS in action. Believers are achievers.

> Consistent positive self-talk is unquestionably one of the greatest gifts to one's subconscious mind.
> —Edmond Mbiaka

Key Points

- Breathe.
- Identify what you would like to invite into your life.
- Retrain your brain by affirming and visualizing the life you want. Imagine what it will feel like when your dreams manifest.
- Keep your thoughts and actions focused on what you want to attract and away from what you don't want. Notice, acknowledge, and dismiss negativity, including envy and insecurity.
- Be open and receptive.
- Expand your knowledge with articles, books, audios, and videos from guides who realized their dreams.
- Surround yourself with kindred spirits and experience the synergy of positive energy as you motivate and encourage one another.
- Ask, take action, believe, and gratefully receive.

Abundance is not something we acquire.
It is something we tune into.
—Wayne Dyer

Now you have your homework to do! Your understanding of the power of your beliefs will help you set your compass to guide you to accomplishing your desires. As you align your positive thoughts and actions, you know that a fulfilling life is available to you. What you think about, and give thanks about, you bring about. The more you have, the more you have to share. Follow your dreams.

CHAPTER 27

Redefine Rejection

Rejection is merely a redirection; a course
correction to your destiny.
—Bryant McGill

Everyone experiences rejection. Experiences can range in intensity from a common one, such as being left out of a group photograph or excluded from a social event, to painful ones, such as being rejected by a loved one. Your perception of rejection and the way you choose to respond will greatly influence the quality of your life.

Research indicates that rejection and physical pain share common neural territory. fMRI (functional magnetic resonance imaging) studies show that the same areas of the brain become activated when we experience rejection as when we experience physical pain. This might explain why a broken heart hurts so much.

We allow rejection to lower our self-esteem when we react to a romantic rejection by finding reasons to blame ourselves, magnify our flaws, and berate ourselves when we are already downhearted. On the other hand, if we determine that there are factors that are too daunting to overcome and we are working too hard to make the relationship mutually beneficial, it becomes easier to accept rejection and move forward.

Adaptable people use rejection to improve and continue in the direction of their dream.

The Beatles are an example of a famous group that persevered despite multiple rejections. In 1962, they auditioned for their first major label on New Year's Day, an opportunity set up by their newly hired manager, Brian Epstein. Despite performing fifteen songs in just under an hour, including three originals, their audition for Decca Records was rejected. Epstein, a man known for his persistence, kept pushing to reverse the label's decision. Decca responded to Epstein's follow-up request by telling him that "guitar groups are on their way out." Decca was not the only label to reject the Beatles; so did Philips, Pye, and Columbia. The Beatles moved past these rejections into international stardom.

You can be more objective when you understand that rejection reflects the other person's perception. You can question whether it was based on logic and wisdom, or if it was an expression of ignorance, prejudice, or other bias. Taking the time to think it through will influence your response to each rejection.

Most fears of rejection rest on the desire for approval from other people. Don't base your self-esteem on their opinions.
—Harvey Mackay

There are several famous artists who were devastated by rejection. The following true story is a good example.

Sergei Rachmaninoff (1873–1943) was a Russian pianist, conductor, and composer. He was trained at the Moscow Conservatory as a pianist, but from youth, his passion was for composition. In 1897, he presented his First Symphony, his most finely constructed work at the time, at the St. Petersburg Conservatory. The reception was a disaster; in fact, the work was compared to a musical representation of hell and the ten plagues of Egypt.

At the time, Rachmaninoff believed that his incompetence was to blame. The unexpected rejection plunged him into a four-year depression. Eventually, after a series of auto-suggestive therapy sessions with a psychiatrist, Rachmaninoff was finally able to restore his self-confidence. He went on to compose what is perhaps his most renowned work: the Second Piano Concerto.

Interestingly enough, historical review later revealed that the excessive criticism had nothing to do with the composition itself but may have been the result of social factors: deep-seated rivalry between the Moscow and St. Petersburg Conservatories; under-rehearsal; and during the performance, the conductor was drunk.

When you become dispassionate about rejection, it won't propel you into self-blame and low self-worth. Activate the curiosity to explore the rejection from a detached perspective to seek clarity.

Here is a story that illustrates how rejection can impact well-being.

Katherine sat in silence as she tried to grasp what her husband, Cedric, had said. After thirty-five years, he needed to put himself first and explore a new life, free of the burdens of a wife and children. He had sublet an apartment, and he was all set to move in that afternoon. Katherine's immediate thoughts were, *I knew this would happen someday. I'm not good enough. He has never loved me, no matter how hard I tried.* Katherine pleaded with Cedric to take some time to think it over and try to work it out. She would change, the children would change, and they would do whatever he wanted them to do.

As Cedric closed the door on his way out, Katherine placed her hand on her aching heart to ease her restricted breathing. Her despair deepened as she ruminated about past rejections, beginning with her high school sweetheart who dumped her when he left for college. Then, the young man in college who would spend hours catching up on his missed classes by sharing her notes but would flirt with her roommate. Finally, her husband, whose family had been unhappy with his choice and had not tried to disguise their disappointment. She kept all this pain trapped in her heart, and she was inconsolable. She believed that only Cedric's return would end her suffering.

The turning point came when their children, who had been angry at being abandoned by Cedric, were now eager to get away from Katherine's depression and hang out with "Dad's cool girlfriend" on the weekends. Katherine sank deeper into isolation. Her fear of rejection became so overwhelming that she repressed her need for human connection. She decided that her only protection would be to reject everyone before they could reject her.

Her doctor pressed her to see the psychotherapist he had recommended. She was apprehensive but agreed that it was time.

Therapy progressed, and Katherine began to look forward to her regular appointments. She was curious where this journey would take her. As she addressed her unresolved issues, she gained insight into her beliefs, feelings, and behaviors. She realized that she had sought safety in the cocoon of isolation and self-pity, unaware of how self-defeating this was. Now, she was committed to learning from the past, releasing all the trapped, negative emotions, and changing her limiting beliefs about rejection. She was acquiring new coping skills that she would access whenever she faced similar situations again. She saw herself emerging like the beautiful monarch butterfly she admired. She looked in the mirror and said, "I'm going to like the new me."

Over the next few months, Katherine's life situation changed as she changed her way of thinking. She made friends and discovered that she could be lighthearted and engaging, and there was life after rejection.

A year later, Cedric called and asked her to meet him for coffee. Katherine realized that when she stopped calling him and begging him to return, she had shifted to self-focus. She listened as Cedric began with little pleasantries. Then he took a breath and told her he was ready to come home. The lease on his apartment was due for renewal, and he was getting a little tired of the bachelor lifestyle. He wanted to be back in his own home with her and the children. Cedric looked at Katherine and noticed how she had changed. She seemed vibrant and relaxed.

Katherine thought about how she had longed to hear those words during her period of depression. Now that she had been working on becoming her own best friend, she was never going back to where she had been. She told him that she loved him and the children missed him, but they would need to explore what each of them wanted in their marriage.

Katherine suggested that they start over and proceed slowly until there was more clarity. Cedric said sharply, "But my lease is up. I have all my stuff packed in the car, and I was planning on moving back home this evening after work."

She responded, "I'm sure you can work it out. I remember the last time you had your stuff packed in the car." She stood up and kissed him lightly on his forehead. She smiled as she walked away, thinking of the times she had used a hairbrush for a microphone as she sang along with Gloria Gaynor's song, "I Will Survive."

Katherine had resolved her past issues and no longer felt abandoned and alone. Time would tell if a respectful, loving relationship was possible for them.

By letting go of the fear of rejection, you gain the internal freedom to make healthy choices. Your self-esteem is no longer dependent on the opinions of other people. Rejection can drive you to make an honest self-evaluation and grow.

> I take rejection as someone blowing a bugle in my ear
> to wake me up and get going, rather than retreat.
> —Sylvester Stallone

This final story is about honoring feelings of rejection and then transforming them into positive action.

Erika had spent more than fifteen years developing a program to serve the needs of college students. From its modest beginning with her and one assistant, the program had grown into an impressive branch of the university, providing psychological and social assistance to students and the community. She approached her superiors to extend the program to include legal assistance. She then hired a young attorney with disabilities, who, she felt, would inspire others. This expansion was so successful that the decision was made to create a new position of director to oversee the entire program. Erika applied, assured that she would be the obvious choice.

A meeting was scheduled to announce the new appointment, and staff and faculty assembled to receive the news. Erika sat in subdued anticipation. Finally, the announcement was made. They had given the position to the young attorney. Erika inhaled sharply, certain that this was a bad dream. She felt a sharp pain in her back like a knife wound. There was silence as all eyes turned to her. She breathed and firmly suppressed her thoughts and feelings. It all seemed surreal as she walked over and congratulated the new director. She excused herself and left the campus to run errands. She was grateful for this temporary escape.

Upon her return to campus, Erika kept repeating the

acronym WAIT (Why Am I Talking) in her mind (chapter 3). She listened quietly as coworkers stopped by to share their shock and disbelief. She survived the agonizingly long day and left for home. Mercifully, this was the Friday before the Memorial Day weekend. She breathed in the security of her home and collapsed on the couch.

She visualized walking up to her boss and throwing her letter of resignation in his face. She fantasized ways she could sabotage the new director. She sobbed at the injustice of having her "baby" ripped from her arms and given to a stranger, while she was cast aside. Rejection, despair, victimhood, and old pain erupted like a volcano. She remembered her father's comments that her brother was the smart one, her sister was the pretty one, and Erika was the nerdy one. She thought about having to work harder in school because of her learning disability.

Erika spent the long weekend lamenting this incredible loss. Her close friends took turns stopping by to provide food, support, and Kleenex. Eventually, she reminded herself that she had a choice. She could remain bitter and defeated or cut her losses and focus on any potential gain. She found it easier to move past rejection when she accepted that everything does not have to have an explanation.

On Monday night, her friends came over and danced around with coordinated hand movements as they sang the lyrics of their rallying song, "I get knocked down, but I get up again. You are never gonna keep me down." They dissolved into laughter, validated her distress, saluted her courage, and assured her she would be okay.

Tuesday morning arrived, and Erika was prepared for her Oscar-winning performance as the undeterred heroine. She greeted everyone in her usual cheerful manner and went to her office. She continued to do her best to contribute to the wonderful program she had built. She decided that her achievement was rewarding, but it would no longer define her.

Word spread throughout the industry that a new employee had taken over Erika's program. Erika's dignified and professional handling of the situation had revealed her self-confidence and fortitude. Six months later, a larger organization approached Erika to apply for an opening that occurred when the managing director retired. Erika was amazed at the turn of events. Had this offer been made earlier, she would have missed this opportunity because of her loyalty to her program. Now that she was unencumbered, she could step up to a new chapter of professional growth. By transforming the sting of rejection into acceptance, she had remained hopeful until there was an outcome far better than she could have imagined.

> If we will be quiet and ready enough, we shall
> find compensation in every disappointment.
> —Henry David Thoreau

Consider also, what happens when you are the one doing the rejecting. There may be any number of reasons, such as declining an invitation, a job applicant, a stressful friendship, or an incompatible relationship. Keep in mind the other person's feelings and plan ahead what you are going to say. Check your motive to ensure that there is no harm intended—for example, retaliation. Identify your emotional state; if there is anger or fear, stabilize yourself first, watch your tone and timing, and proceed only from a calm, caring place. Choose honest, descriptive, factual, sensitive words. Observe the other person's reaction quietly and refrain from being pulled into an argument. Listen with curiosity and think before you speak. Be respectful and considerate.

Key Points

- Breathe.
- Accept that everyone experiences rejection.
- Acknowledge emotions, surrender, and release.
- Challenge and replace any negative perception of rejection.
- Learn and grow.
- Tap into your inner strength.
- Repeat helpful phrases to keep you strong.
- Reach out for compassionate social support.
- Check your intention, tone, and timing when you are doing the rejecting.
- Gain self-confidence and wisdom.

With each rejection, you have the choice to respond one way or another. Redefine rejection to create the shift in consciousness that will allow you to apply healthy coping skills and strengthen your resolve to live in acceptance and peace. Use tools from pervious chapters, such as reframing, not taking things personally, and self-care, to safeguard your well-being. Relax, reflect, and enjoy the journey.

CHAPTER 28

Live in the Present Moment

> Every morning we are born again. What
> we do today is what matters most.
> —Jack Kornfield

The mind seems to be constantly trying to escape the present moment by identifying with the past or future. In this fast-paced world, you may pack an activity into every waking moment, feeling compelled to always be doing something. The mind is your valuable resource. Do you take time to look after your mind? When was the last time you spent five or ten minutes doing nothing? This means a break from everything: reading, watching television, using your cell phone or computer, or any other activities.

Making time to simply be in the moment may seem contrary to beliefs about the habits of the high achiever. As we get more and more stressed with deadlines, we are forced to prioritize. Often we cut back on rest and stress-relieving techniques and replace them with more stressors. Our bodies react by giving us wake-up calls in the form of accidents or illnesses. We can pay attention to these signals or override them with rationalizations or medication. Coming down with a cold, take two pills and keep on going; backache, take painkillers and keep on doing whatever it was that injured your back in the first place. The signals get louder and louder, and one day we are surprised that we are lying in a hospital bed with pneumonia or facing back surgery. Then we call it bad luck.

Now the new message is "work smart, not hard" or the law of diminishing results, when tasks take longer and are done less efficiently because we have pushed ourselves beyond reasonable limits.

> I have so much to accomplish today that I must
> meditate for two hours instead of one.
> —Mahatma Gandhi

Living in the present moment is discovering that timeless space where you accept that life is unfolding now. This is mindfulness, which is enhanced by calming the mind's endless chatter. Create the practice of making time to sit in silence, embracing the stillness, connecting with your higher self and being grateful and peaceful, watching thoughts come and go without judgment. Make the commitment to do this every day, to recharge your emotional, physical, and spiritual well-being. This will allow you to be in the eternal present and use the past or future when necessary to contribute to improving your life situation. Be patient. Be in this moment, not distracted by the next one. It is always the precious, present moment.

> Today I'll live in the moment, unless it's
> unpleasant, in which case I'll eat a cookie.
> —The Cookie Monster

Your next questions may be "How do I begin? Where can I begin?" There are simple techniques that can be incorporated in daily activities. For example, as you take your shower in the privacy of your own bathroom, focus on the experience of cleansing your body while thinking of the word *flow*. Be acutely aware of every sensation: feeling the water against your skin, the smell and texture of the soap, the sight and sound of the falling water. By thinking or saying the word *flow*, you keep your attention on the experience. To make this even more meaningful, imagine that you had been in the dry, harsh, sandy desert for days, where there was barely enough drinking water. This stark picture would create a greater appreciation for something as simple as taking a shower. You would be able to experience the symbolism of cleansing mind, body, and spirit. Many religions have rituals about cleansing, and this technique provides a simple method to stay focused on the present moment.

You can extend the practice of mindfulness to other ordinary activities, for example putting gas in your car. I could remember the times when other drivers would honk their horns to alert me about the gas tank cover dangling on the side of my car. I decided to change my habit of trying to do multiple tasks simultaneously, like replacing the gas tank cover while the receipt was being printed, by breaking this task down into individual steps. I committed to paying attention to each step, from taking the key out of the ignition and accessing my credit card all the way to deliberately putting the receipt and credit card back into my wallet. Each action from the moment I pulled into the gas station until I drove away became an opportunity to be completely focused. This required perhaps three additional minutes, and the reward was I felt peaceful as I drove away, without having to worry that I had forgotten to do one thing or the other. I felt vital instead of stressed, as if I had taken a mini time-out.

In the East, this is referred to as the state of pure consciousness. Now, whenever I find myself wondering whether I locked the door or when I have to run back to pick up something I left behind, I interpret this as a slowdown message to breathe deeply and give myself the gift of the present moment. Great examples are the avid beekeepers who experience calming and peaceful present-moment awareness as they lovingly tend their bees.

Society placed high regard on multitasking; the person who raced through life, juggling several things simultaneously, was admired. As the resulting stress escalates, so does the pressure on mind, body, and spirit, accompanied by feelings of frustration, impatience, and irritation. Multitasking is now more appropriately labeled "techno stress."

Silence is a wonderful doorway to the present moment. Thich Nhat Hanh, in his book *Peace Is Every Step*, has a wonderful idea about having a "breathing room" in your home, a place where you can enter with the guarantee not to be disturbed. This is your sanctuary, with perhaps a little bell that lets you and everyone know you are breathing and restoring your peace. Your caring loved one is welcome to join you in the nurturing silence. Perhaps you cannot have an entire room, so you have a closet dedicated to this purpose or the corner of a room with symbolic items, like flowers, statues, or paintings.

Meditation can enhance peace in the present moment, and there are many types of meditation that can be easily incorporated in daily living. People who have a meditation practice show less cortisol release (the harmful hormone released by the hypothalamus, which induces stress) and lower levels of anxiety, depression, anger, and fatigue. Interestingly enough, I found a method of meditation when I was floating in a swimming pool, looking up at the sky, feeling relaxed and grateful. This prompted me to write the following poem, my first published work, "Floating":

> Floating in the ocean
> arms and legs resting on the waves

like a limp X
as I watch the clouds tell their story.
I feel so peaceful
and in harmony with nature,
all is well in my world
and I am content.
How can I extend this feeling
into my daily routine
balancing turmoil with tranquility
keeping things in perspective.
It all seems so simple
floating here in the ocean
a sweet sense of surrender
a time to retreat and replenish.

There was a similar experience after Susan installed a hammock in a covered area in her backyard. As she was lying in the hammock, Susan felt deeper peace and present-moment awareness. The next day, her little daughter, Baili, joined her in the hammock and this began a daily practice of taking a time-out from all distractions to nurture their souls and their connection.

Mindfulness meditation is the moment in which you are fully conscious and connected with the present moment. Ram Dass wrote of being in a monastery and watching a monk who was fully focused on the dish he was washing. Jessica shared about filling a glass with water, listening to the sound of the water, watching it rise slowly, and feeling the coolness of the glass as it frosted on the outside.

Present-moment awareness can be brought to every activity. For example, have you rushed through a meal so unconsciously that you were oblivious of the taste, aroma, and presentation? In Jamaica, this is referred to as "*nam* and scram," when someone gobbles down his food and dashes off immediately afterward. This mindless consumption often comes with a generous side dish of gastric distress. Slowing down to appreciate each bite enriches the dining experience. There is a heightened sense of replenishing the body, along with gratitude to all who made this food available. For example, you bless the farmer who harvested the delicious vegetables on your plate.

Mindfulness keeps us from going into auto pilot, and
each moment is lived fully, a moment not to be missed.
—Unknown

Consider the golden eagle, soaring across the blue sky, wings extended. The golden eagle isn't thinking about the squirrel he did not catch earlier that morning with thoughts such as, *Gosh, I should have made more of an effort to catch that squirrel. I am beginning to feel hungry. I missed a good opportunity.* The golden eagle is also not thinking, *What if there are no more squirrels? I could starve to death. I'm not like the sea eagles that prefer eating fish.*

The golden eagle is completely in the here and now, gliding effortlessly at great heights. With his remarkable eyesight, five times sharper than humans, if he suddenly spots a prey, he'll swoop down, catch and consume it, all in the present moment. Perhaps the golden eagle is inviting you to be more mindfully present by going from "nowhere" to "now here."

Some people feel the rain, others just get wet.
Embracing the present moment is a way to
live in harmony with impermanence.
—Roger Miller

Key Points

- Breathe.
- Take time-outs for calming meditation.
- Use everyday activities to practice mindfulness.
- Be here now. Catch yourself when you drift aimlessly into the past or fast-forward to the future.
- Live your life as a moment-to-moment experience.
- Make the best use of today.

The essence of a new day:

> This is the beginning of a new day. You have been given this day to use as you will. You can waste it or use it for good. What you do today is important because you are exchanging a day of your life for it. When tomorrow comes, this day will be gone forever; in its place is something that you have left behind ... let it be something good. —Unknown

Find that delicate balance. Spend just enough time in the past to learn from your successes and failures. Think about the future just long enough to prepare for it. Knowing that your point of power is the present moment, redirect your focus from "what was" or "what if" to "what is," mindful of what you hear, see, and feel.

Make a habit of spending most of your time in the present, motivated by the realization that everything is temporary and love is all there is. Each precious moment cannot be replaced. When asked what her thoughts were on death, an elder responded, "One day you'll die, but the rest of the days you won't." With many days behind her, she was not about to waste the present moment; she celebrates living now. How about you?

CHAPTER 29

Be Peaceful

World Peace begins with Inner Peace.
—Dalai Lama

The path to inner peace begins with the understanding that peace is within you, aligned with the popular saying that you are "a human being, not a human doing." There will be moments when you find it easier to access this peace than at other times. Reflect on that quiet place deep in the lake, away from the turmoil on the surface, to mentally retreat and replenish. Seek the clarity of a calm mind, free from endless thinking, like clearing out a room crammed with unnecessary clutter.

With all the discord across the nation and the world, it becomes increasingly important to notice when negativity seeps into conversations and invades your thoughts. There are many issues that can pull you into the cacophony of chaos, when you are triggered to descend into the lower-frequency emotions of fear, anger, envy, hate, and judgment. The saying "peace of mind comes piece by piece" would suggest that it is a moment-to-moment choice to be peaceful.

As the compassionate observer, you become an agent of peace. With loving detachment, you determine if and how you can help without being overwhelmed and fearful. There is a time for appropriate action, and there is a time to refrain from action. You aspire to be a part of the peaceful solution.

Strengthen your inner peace with a disciplined focus on feeding your mind, soul, and body with healthy nourishment, along with uplifting physical activities such as breathing, stretching, and walking. Make time for regular meditation. Reinforce your peacefulness with readings or videos, prayer, positive ideas, and humor.

The intention of being peaceful becomes a compass to guide you through all the events that unfold. Occasions when you are triggered to give up your peace, you stop and reset your compass to find your way back to peace.

It isn't enough to talk about peace. One must believe in it.
And it isn't enough to believe in it. One must work at it.
—Eleanor Roosevelt

This story is about recognizing challenges to peace. Mike and Elizabeth had experienced many trials and tribulations with their only son. As the consequences of his behaviors escalated, they were often tense and guarded. With consistent effort and professional help, they became a team and made inner peace their first priority. They accepted that there would be times when they needed to step aside and allow their son to find his own way.

One evening, as Mike was preparing for a business trip, Elizabeth sensed his growing unrest. Their son had gone out for the evening, and he was later than usual coming home. Elizabeth refrained from her old behavior of calling and texting their son frantically in order to alleviate Mike's fears. She took deep breaths and tried to remain detached. Their unspoken words hung heavily between them. When their son came home, he acknowledged being late and happily shared with them all about his evening. He looked at them and hesitated momentarily, perhaps feeling the unspoken tension. He wished them a good night and left for bed.

The next morning as they were heading for the airport, Elizabeth took this time to invite Mike to share his thoughts about the previous evening. Upon reflection, Mike recognized that he had muffled his concerns about his business trip. He had unconsciously shifted his focus to the familiar unease he felt whenever their son was late. Elizabeth said, "I felt us giving away our peace by going back to the old distressful pattern. Later I pondered the question, *Where was God in the equation?*" They both reflected on this poignant question. They were reminded of the vigilance required to safeguard peace by replacing fear with prayer.

This often-told Taoist story illustrates the value of maintaining your peace despite outer circumstances. There was an old farmer who had worked his crops for many years.

One day his horse ran away. Upon hearing the news, his neighbors came to visit. "Such bad luck," they said sympathetically."

"Maybe," the farmer replied.

The next morning, the horse returned, bringing with it three other wild horses. "How wonderful!" the neighbors exclaimed."

Maybe," replied the old man.

The following day, his son tried to ride one of the untamed horses, was thrown, and broke his leg. The neighbors again came to offer their sympathy on his misfortune. "Maybe," answered the farmer.

The following day, military officials came to the village to draft young men into the army. Seeing that the son's leg was broken, they passed him by. The neighbors congratulated the farmer on how well things had turned out. "Maybe," said the farmer.

When you look at experiences as they are and understand

that everything passes, you learn to maintain your peace. You get off the roller-coaster ride of reacting to the ups and downs, and you breathe out stressful thoughts and feelings. With a clear mind, you are able to determine the next appropriate step.

Intriguing research illustrated that as a direct result of a large group practicing meditation, violence in the surrounding area decreased significantly. The meditators affirmed that love was more powerful than fear. They believed in the power of collective energy to bring healing to the world.

When you walk beyond the wall of fear and separateness, you get in touch with your compassionate inner self and experience internal transformation. You wake up individually and contribute to the awakening of the world, free of the restrictions of race, gender, religion, socioeconomic status, and so on. Believing that at the deepest level we are all one, you see yourself as part of the global community, striving to build a more compassionate society. No longer separate, you want the highest good for everyone, and you wake up collectively.

There is also the influential effect of music. Many of our youth have been motivated to make significant life changes by having their musical talents channeled through inspirational music. There are personal stories of young people who felt the despair of heading in the wrong direction and experiencing the escalating consequences of poor choices. These troubled young people reversed their downward spiral after attending a youth group or concert and hearing others share a similar path to disgrace and their empowering U-turn to grace. These artists have carried on the legacy of influencing countless other people to apply their talents to peaceful goals. Positive tone and lyrics have encouraged people to participate in their community, their country, and other parts of the world.

Music is also a unifying expression of culture and heritage, as traditions are passed on from one generation to the other. Hearing a familiar refrain has often brought nostalgia to someone who left their ancestral home, bringing a feeling of connection and shared history. Social media has opened new possibilities of contacting distant relatives and dissolving barriers to peaceful, global connection.

The regional chamber of commerce, the New England Council, had a thoughtful slogan: "A rising tide lifts all the boats." John F. Kennedy often borrowed this slogan. The phrase was used more commonly to defend tax cuts. It seemed like a good idea to borrow this slogan and apply it a little differently. Envision a world in which positive, peaceful thinkers would connect energetically from all parts of the world, and this rising tide of peaceful intention would lift other thinkers and help them shed the heavy weight of negativity. Each decision would be guided by the question "What would love do here?"

Each time you affirm one peaceful thought, you are part of the positive shift. Nothing has to change for you to be peaceful. You can embrace inner peace anytime, anywhere.

Many have strengthened their commitment to peace by regularly reciting a version of the loving kindness meditation.

The first time you use "I" for self– focus. The second time you use "You" and picture someone you care about. The third time you use "They" and include family, friends, neighbors in your country and the world.

> May I be filled with loving kindness.
> May I be well,
> May I be peaceful and at ease.
> May I be happy.
> May I live in peace no matter what is given to me.

When inner peace blesses your life and contributes to world peace, you discover that each time you send love to the person in front of you, you can make a difference to that person. This concept is reflected in that often-told story "The Star Thrower" by Loren Eiseley.

> While wandering a deserted beach at dawn, stagnant in my work, I saw a man in the distance bending and throwing as he walked the open stretch toward me. As he came near, I could see that he was throwing starfish, abandoned on the sand by the tide, back into the sea. When he was close enough I asked him why he was working so hard at this strange task. He said that the sun would dry the starfish and they would die. I told him that I thought he was foolish. There were thousands of starfish on miles and miles of beach. One man alone could never make a difference. He smiled as he picked up the next starfish. Hurling it far into the sea he said, "It makes a difference for this one." I abandoned my writing and spent the morning throwing starfish.

You may never know the impact of a kind word spoken at a pivotal time in another person's life. Each time you strengthen your role of peacemaker, you have an opportunity to be an integral part of a peaceful world, one starfish at a time.

You can be an instrument of peace, with God as the conductor of the orchestra. Each peaceful thought or action contributes to the energy of the planet. This gives you a great responsibility to be mindful of your thoughts and actions as they impact the environment. A smile is a great way to spread the "infection" of positive energy.

Smiling is very important. If we are not able
to smile the world will not have peace.
—Thich Nhat Hanh

Beth had this opportunity to impart peace in a casual interaction at the airport. She was awaiting the arrival of her sister's flight. A confused tourist approached Beth and asked in halting English for directions to baggage claim. They chatted briefly, and Beth guided the tourist to the escalator and wished her a wonderful vacation in Miami or wherever her travels would take her. The relieved tourist thanked Beth and hurried off to locate her luggage. In those few minutes, Beth's helpful response created that tourist's first positive impression of Miami and the United States of America. Beth was the US ambassador of first impressions.

I made labels for the envelopes of all outgoing mail, "Peace in all hearts." The license plate on my car is "B PCEFUL." Often drivers will wave at me with a thumbs-up, and people stop by my car to validate the message. I've had people pass by my office and say, "I'm sure that must be your car in the parking lot with the peaceful license plate." This spills over into every encounter I have, and I seem to run into peaceful people often.

This is a story about making peace a priority. Michael and Sheryl had gone to pick up a rental car. They were in a hurry because they were running behind on completing many other tasks before heading out on a road trip. Sheryl was becoming exasperated by the painfully slow process. She glanced over at Michael, surprised that he appeared to be so calm.

As if responding to her unspoken question, Michael looked directly at Sheryl and asked, "What is your purpose in life?"

The question seemed so out of sync with her agitation that she frowned at him and said, "I don't know. I guess to be kind."

He paused and then said, "Your purpose in life is to get closer to God."

Sheryl stopped for a moment and received this insight as a priceless gift. Suddenly everything seemed so clear. Was this silly experience worth jeopardizing her inner peace? Was anything worth jeopardizing inner peace? She thanked Michael for being her *upa* guru. Upa Guru means the teacher nearby who shows you part of the way. The next time that you face a difficult situation, determine how to make inner peace your first priority.

> Anything that costs you your peace is too expensive.
> —Unknown

Take your role as peacemaker very seriously. Use every encounter to plant seeds of peace and hope. Begin by planting the seeds within. Thus, you strengthen the peace and grace inside, which radiates outward to other people. Marian shared her prescription—Rx for peace, GOD: gratitude, optimism, detachment.

There is a cute story about a restless king who looked for a man who slept well. He hoped to buy his bed, only to learn that the man had no bed, but he had peace.

Key Points

- Breathe.

- Make time for peace reinforcing activities such as meditation.
- Look for opportunities to promote peace.
- Identify the issue that is threatening your peace.
- Decline the invitation to participate in the chaos.
- Ask, "Am I willing to give up my peace for this?"
- Apply the appropriate tools for each situation.
- Choose peace over fear.

Imagine all the people living life in peace.
You may say I'm a dreamer, but I'm not the only one.
I hope someday you'll join us, and the world will be as one.
—John Lennon

Moment to moment, you have the choice to claim your power and be a peaceful influence or to give away your power by reacting negatively. You get this opportunity all the time, on the highways and byways, with loved ones, in stores or offices. Every contact gives you the chance to pass on a positive message, verbally or nonverbally. Imagine a world in which every person committed to being an instrument of peace. Embrace the words from that beautiful hymn, "Let there be peace on earth, and let it begin with me."

CHAPTER 30

Be Grateful

The most direct route to well-being is Gratitude.

The previous guidelines/tools overlap and reinforce one another, with gratitude as a common thread. Thus, gratitude is the antidote for everything. An interesting article suggested that focusing on gratitude can shut down the part of the brain that worries. Like other activities such as physical exercise, practicing feeling and expressing gratitude can be seen as strengthening your brain muscle. The more you practice, the more automatic this becomes.

It is exciting to see the mainstream health practices' approach to well-being move beyond simply the physical and incorporate the concept of mind, body, spirit. Recent research is exploring the impact of higher-frequency emotions such as gratitude on health. Expressions of gratitude release endorphins into the bloodstream, thereby enhancing the immune system, which in turn makes you more resistant to disease and even speeds up the recovery process. This release of endorphins also stimulates dilation of the blood vessels, which in turn leads to a relaxed heart. Consider that you benefit each time you say "thank you" for even the smallest kindness, in addition to validating the other person.

If the only prayer you ever say in your entire
life is thank you, it will be enough.
—Meister Eckhart

Look for articles and studies to reinforce your commitment to being grateful. According to Emmons's research, grateful people—those who perceive gratitude as a permanent trait rather than a temporary state of mind—have an edge on the not-so-grateful when it comes to health. "Grateful people take better care of themselves and engage in more protective health behaviors like regular exercise, a healthy diet, regular physical examinations," said University of California Davis psychology professor Robert Emmons.

Bracket each day with gratitude thoughts. Set the tone for a positive interpretation of the day's unfolding. Upon awakening, the first conscious thought would be a reflection on a reason to be grateful, thereby short-circuiting the stress thoughts that can automatically come up. Throughout the day, being mindful of every positive interaction and using each opportunity to express gratitude can significantly enhance life satisfaction. At the end of each day, you would have the closing bracket after reviewing and expressing gratitude for all the blessings and lessons you have received. This would certainly be a healthy alternative to watching the late-night news. Your subconscious will play your last thoughts all through the night.

Each day we are given 86,000 seconds. How
many of these do we use being grateful?
—Adapted from several sources

Several motivators recommend the strategy of creating a gratitude list. This gives you a visual reminder of the good things that you may otherwise take for granted. As you add items to the list, your capacity for gratitude expands. For example, whenever you pay attention to your gift of sight, colors become more vibrant, the butterfly appears more beautiful and graceful.

This story of appreciation is about a young man, Harry, who had undergone eye surgery with an uncertain outcome. As Harry approached the day when his bandages would be removed, he reminded himself that he would accept the outcome without fear, believing that his medical team had done everything possible to restore his sight. Slowly the bandages were removed, and he was instructed to keep his eyes closed. He was led out onto the patio and asked to gradually open his eyes. He took a deep breath and began to slowly open his eyes, experiencing the sensation of moving from darkness to light. Almost in disbelief, he began to observe outlines. Within minutes, he gasped at the range of vibrant colors of the afternoon sunset. Harry looked around this beautiful setting and asked, "Where is everybody?" How was it possible, he thought, that he alone stood there in awe of this panorama? When was the last time you paused to appreciate the beauty of nature?

A grateful heart is a magnet for miracles.
—*Inspirational Heart* magazine

This story is about being grateful for what you have rather than brooding over what you lost. There is a young woman named Jackie who had a tumor removed from her brain. The surgery saved her life, but she lost her sense of smell. This was initially seen as a small price to pay, especially by her parents, who had lost her older brother, also to a brain tumor, just two years prior.

Jackie learned that her sense of smell was necessary not only for protection but also for digestion, memory, emotions, and motor skills, such as maintenance of balance. Because taste and smell are intimately linked, when she lost her sense of smell, she also lost her appetite. While she was assured that her taste buds were still working and would still detect sweet, sour, bitter, and salty, without the olfactory cells in the nose that allowed her to appreciate the delicious complexities of flavor, each meal became as appetizing as vaguely seasoned newspaper.

Prior to her surgery, Jackie had not given any thought to her sense of smell, and she found that people in general did not rank the sense of smell very high. Yet in the early stage when she realized that she would be deprived of the sensual pleasure of eating and drinking, she found herself drifting into depression. This was compounded when she noticed that she was also having problems with balance. When she learned that one in twenty people are affected with anosmia, as it is called, she realized that she would have to learn how to cope with this loss.

She battled her way from self-pity to acceptance and then moved forward to gratitude for her life and for her other senses. She relied on memory to recapture the smells she had lost, and she reengaged in the act of living. She became a living example of the importance of gratitude and the life-changing impact of being grateful every moment. Rather than pining for the sense she had lost, she became more grateful for the ones she had left. Colors became brighter, sounds sweeter, and she had a heightened awareness of touch. Every time she went to a concert, she looked and listened with a higher level of appreciation. She reflected on all the things she had previously taken for granted.

Give thanks for unknown blessings already on their way.
—Native American prayer

There's an old saying, "If you've forgotten the language of gratitude, you'll never be on speaking terms with happiness." It's wise to give this serious consideration. Several studies have shown depression to be inversely correlated to gratitude. It seems that the more grateful a person is, the less depressed they are. Philip Watkins, a clinical psychologist at Eastern Washington University, found that clinically depressed individuals showed significantly lower levels of gratitude (nearly 50 percent less) than nondepressed controls.

> It is impossible to feel grateful and
> depressed in the same moment.
> —Naomi Williams

However, when depressed feelings arise, it is unproductive to chastise yourself because you "should" not be having these feelings when you have so much you "should" be grateful for. With this thinking, you end up feeling worse.

Instead, identify and honor the feelings, then gently release and replace them with gratitude for an aspect of your life. Become more grateful for all that you learn from coping with challenging people and situations. Ensure that your self-talk is positive, encouraging, and appreciative. This eventually becomes a healthy habit of self-kindness and understanding, using gratitude to restore well-being.

Another caution is to let go of any expectations of being thanked for your kind act. Your reward comes from passing on the gifts that were given to you, and any expression of appreciation from the other person is a bonus. This frees you from any negativity when giving or receiving. Justine remembered the special present she had given a dear friend at her birthday celebration. Two days later, Justine's friend called to say thank you, because she was not sure if she had told Justine how much she liked her gift. Justine was pleasantly surprised and happy that she had not tarnished the gift with any negative thoughts.

This story illustrates the attitude of gratitude. Two boys were like brothers, except that Christian came from an underprivileged family, and Edward came from a wealthy, prestigious home. It was ironic to see that Edward remained envious of the materially poor Christian, because he could never experience gratitude. On one occasion, Christian was happy with his gift of a whistle. In contrast, Edward felt no pleasure with the beautiful pony his father had gotten him, and he was irritated by what he considered to be Christian's stupid joy. Edward thought it was ridiculous to be excited about a silly whistle, whereas Christian had the ability to extract joy from everything.

Later in the story, when Christian achieved great wealth, this did not become the measure of his happiness. He had already determined that happiness is inside. He had learned from a wise guide that "Your circumstances do not determine your possibilities. When you shift your perception through a daily gratitude practice, you condition your mind for abundance."

> A grateful attitude becomes the grid
> through which you perceive life.
> —From *Jesus Calling*

Eric Butterworth, in his seminal book *Spiritual Economics,* provides a thought-provoking concept regarding money. This could stimulate a shift in consciousness. "Never allow money of any kind or amount to pass through your hands without blessing it, whether it is coming to you or going from you ... Keep the awareness that it is currency, a movement of divine flow. When it comes to you, give thanks that it has flowed from the infinite through your job or investment. When it goes from you, give thanks that there is no depletion, but actually increase because you have kept it flowing."

This final story shows the value of realizing how blessed you are for everything you have. This can be challenging at certain times, as was the case in the story of two families in California. After a devastating fire that destroyed an entire town, the press interviewed an elderly couple who kept lamenting, "We lost everything, we lost everything." It was unsettling to witness their despair.

Later that afternoon, the microphone was given to another couple as they looked in disbelief at the rubble that had been their home. They said, "We lost everything material, our home, our possessions of a lifetime, and we felt overwhelmed. Now we pause and realize that everything that is irreplaceable is absolutely perfect: our children, our pets, each other, and we are filled with gratitude." The immediate reaction was similar for both couples. The second couple, by accessing inner strength and gratitude, was able to return their focus to everything they had left, and their spirits were uplifted.

> Gratitude is a soil in which Joy thrives.
> —Berthold Auerbach

Key Points

- Breathe.
- Use brackets to begin and end each day with gratitude thoughts.
- Remind yourself that gratitude opens the path to abundance.
- Look for reasons to express your gratitude.

- Gratitude is the antidote for everything. Use it for attitude adjustment.
- Be open and receptive to all the good.

The secret to a long and healthy life is to be stress-free.
Be grateful for everything you have, stay away from
people who are negative, stay smiling and keep running.
—Fanja Singh, hundred-year-old marathoner

Gratitude enhances emotional, mental, physical and spiritual well-being. It activates your subconscious to show you reasons to be grateful. When gratitude is your default mode, you intentionally look for the hidden blessings in every situation. Switching the attention from lack to gratitude fosters abundance. Ultimately, you see this as an invaluable resource, and you are grateful that you have the capacity to experience gratitude in each moment.

CHAPTER 31

Bring Back Joy

"Joy does not simply happen to us. We have to
choose joy and keep choosing it every day."
—Henri J. M. Nouwen

At the end of each Wednesday group, we recite the mantra "Acceptance, wellness, bringing back joy," followed by "The circle of love begins with me." This propels the participants to go forth and live each day in joy with the understanding that you can enlarge your capacity for joy. Thus, *Bring Back Joy* seemed like a fitting title for this final chapter.

Marie's story illustrates how any burden you have been carrying becomes lighter when you discover that sadness and joy can coexist and enrich each other. There can be appreciation for the sunshine after rainy days and the rain after a long drought.

Marie had not been able to enjoy her older son's successful promotion while her younger son was experiencing the debilitating consequences of substance abuse. Often siblings feel robbed of their parents' attention because of all the energy focused on the child with the problem. Consciously or unconsciously, their resentment builds toward the "problem child," as if they did not already have enough to deal with.

It is helpful to contemplate one of the 12 Laws of Karma, "One cannot focus on good and bad at the same time." The

269

object of your focus will determine your enjoyment in the moment, without detracting from any actions you may need to take at the appropriate time. Marie could enjoy her older son's success and also be available to support her younger son's path to recovery. Thus she would love both sons unconditionally, sharing their accomplishments and their challenges.

> Talking about our problems is our greatest
> addiction. Break the habit. Talk about your joys.
> —Rita Schiano

Jack became tearful as he expressed his wish that he had learned this concept of being open to joy sooner. He reflected on his painful childhood experiences until his aggressive father passed away and his mother later married the next-door neighbor. When his mother's new husband tried to be the kind father Jack had always wanted, he felt shackled by misguided guilt, as if he were being strangely disloyal to his heartless, unlovable father. Burying his deepest need, he closed his heart to the love offered by his stepfather.

Many years later, Jack learned that a joyful heart has no limits, and there was more than enough room to create a special place in his expanding heart for this good man. He wished he could go back in time and enjoy the love that was being freely offered to him, or at least be able to express his gratitude. Now that both his mother and stepfather had passed away, he committed to honoring them by embracing joy every day and sharing this with his own children. He would not delay a moment longer to experience joy.

> Joy comes to us in ordinary moments, we
> risk missing out on joy when we get too
> busy chasing down the extraordinary.
> —Brené Brown

When each day is welcomed from a joyful perspective, this becomes the filter through which you process everything around you. You can apply the tools from the preceding chapters to guide your life's journey and reinforce all that you learn from other sources. Commit to a peaceful, joyful path, happy to plant seeds along the way to any fellow travelers who will listen and share with you their own wisdom.

If you carry joy in your heart, you can heal any moment.
—Charles Santana

Joy is sustainable under any circumstances when you incorporate messages such as Ecclesiastes 3 (KJV), "To everything there is a season, and a time to every purpose under the heaven." This is further strengthened by the gift of the "faith that surpasses understanding." Life may become joyless during difficult times, when it all feels overwhelming. Laughter is a way to keep joy alive in the midst of sadness.

As three generations gathered around their beloved grandpa on his deathbed, there was a sense of impending loss blended with gratitude that they could all be there with him. With a twinkle in his eye, Grandpa retold his favorite joke, and the room exploded with laughter. Grandpa was able to have his sense of humor right to the end, giving them another precious memory.

Another example is driving west on Kendall Drive in Miami, feeling irritated by the rush hour drivers. At the same time, there is a breathtaking sunset ahead. Since both exist simultaneously, your choice of where to place your attention will result in moments of irritation or joy.

Consider another situation. An overcast sky can seem so gloomy. You look farther and see a break in the dark clouds revealing a small patch of blue. In that moment, you focus on the tiny blue area and smile, remembering blue skies on sunny days. Don't miss pockets of joy! Live in joy through acceptance. A life free of attachment enjoys the present moment and makes no demand that it last.

Here is another example of an event that was reframed to bring joy. I had purchased a fashionable ski jacket for my son, Jamie, for our Thanksgiving ski trip out west. The following winter, there was an unusual cold front at home in Ft. Lauderdale. With temperatures in the low forties, Floridians were "freezing." Jamie called me and said, "Mom, there's something I have to tell you. I hope you won't get mad."

I replied, "Okay."

He continued, "On my way to work, I saw this sweet old lady sitting on the side of the street, shivering and alone. I hurried back home, and the warmest thing I grabbed was that great ski jacket you gave me last year. I took it to her. I hope you don't mind."

In that moment, I inhaled sharply. A brief pause allowed me to reframe my initial thought—*You did what!*—to appreciation of his spontaneous generosity.

Almost a year later, Jamie was in the same area of town, and he noticed someone waving frantically at him. He could not believe his eyes. There was the same little old lady, waving and smiling, showing him that she was still wearing the ski jacket, now several shades darker from a great deal of use. Jamie experienced that wonderful endorphin rush that comes from the joy of giving. We may not have outstanding ways to serve, and so we strive to be joyful through small acts of kindness.

> I expect to pass through this world but once,
> any good thing therefore that I can do,
> or any goodness that I can show to any fellow creature,

let me do it now,
let me not defer or neglect it,
for I shall not pass this way again.
—John Wesley

As you come to the end of this final chapter, hopefully you envision personal change, and you will reinforce all the thoughts and actions that enhance your well-being and promote joy. Writing this book helps me to pass on what I have learned (what "Eye See") and reminds me to practice what I preach. This can be your reference book to make the best of life situations. God is good. He wants us to be good to ourselves and to one another and live joyfully.

Key Points

- Breathe.
- Carry joy in your heart.
- Remember that joy and sadness can coexist.
- Find joy in ordinary moments.
- When outer circumstances threaten your joy, go inside where joy resides.
- Be filled with joy and infect the world.

The object of the Dance is not to finish, it's to dance.
—Michael Mahoney

Your journey becomes a glorious dance as each day unfolds and you continue learning and applying the steps to move gracefully along the dance floor of life. Keep your heart open to all of life's experiences, appreciating what you have, and knowing that you do not need anything, or anyone, to be fulfilled. You are whole and complete, and you are aware of the importance of human connection. May you have a teachable spirit, as you mindfully incorporate these guidelines into your own self-care program and create your path to resilient and joyful living!

Envision a better you and a better world. May you be blessed and be a blessing to others!

Printed in the United States
By Bookmasters